The Thyroid Fix

HOW TO REDUCE FATIGUE, LOSE WEIGHT, AND GET YOUR LIFE BACK

Dr. Shawn Soszka

Evergreen Integrative Medicine, LLC

Portland, Oregon

Shawn Soszka/Evergreen Integrative Medicine, LLC
7215 SE 13th Ave
Portland, Oregon 97202
www.TheThyroidFixBook.com

Editor: Ryan Carrasco
Cover Design: Andrej Semnic aka "Semnitz"
Book Layout: ©2017 BookDesignTemplates.com
Photograph: Kristal Passy Photography

Ordering Information:

Quantity sales. Special discounts are available on quantity purchases by corporations, associations, and others. For details, contact the "Special Sales Department" at the address above.

The Thyroid Fix/ Shawn Soszka. —1st ed.

ISBN 978-1-7321601-1-8

Contents

Free Bonus Videos 13

Introduction 15

    Why I Wrote This Book 15

    Is This Book Right for You? 16

    The Holistic Approach to Thyroid Problems 17

    Who is Dr. Soszka? 18

How the Thyroid Works 21

    Thyroid: The Big Picture 21

    It Starts in the Brain 23

    The Thyroid 24

    How Thyroid Hormone is Transported 25

    Thyroid Hormone Conversion 25

    Thyroid Hormone Receptors and Activation 26

    Chapter Highlights 28

Do You Have Symptoms of Underactive Thyroid? 29

    Common Symptoms of Low Thyroid 29

    Special Focus: Fatigue 33

    Special Focus: Weight Loss 35

Special Focus: Hormone Imbalance 36

Chapter Highlights 39

The Many Causes of Low Thyroid Function 41

Signaling and Feedback Errors in the Brain 42

Thyroid Hormone Conversion Disorders 45

Decreased Thyroid Hormone Conversion 48

Reverse T3 50

Thyroid Hormone Resistance and Receptor Defects 51

Chapter Highlights 54

Hashimoto's Thyroiditis 55

Why Autoimmunity Goes Untreated 56

Your Thyroid is Under Attack! 57

The Causes of Hashimoto's Thyroiditis 59

The Symptoms of Hashimoto's Thyroiditis 62

Special Topics in Hashimoto's Thyroiditis 63

The Iodine Controversy 64

Low-Dose Naltrexone 66

Chapter Highlights 69

Liver, Digestion, and Adrenals 71

Liver Dysfunction and Thyroid Conversion Problems 72

Disease Begins in the Digestive Tract 75

The Role of Intestinal Bacteria in Thyroid Problems 80

Do You Have Parasites or an Intestinal Infection? 81

Adrenal Fatigue Syndrome and Low Thyroid 84

Adrenal Fatigue Syndrome and Chronic Stress 85

Testing for Adrenal Fatigue Syndrome 88

Chapter Highlights 90

Why Thyroid Disorders Are Not Treated Effectively 91

The Narrow Perspective of Conventional Medicine 91

Outdated Mechanical Thinking 92

The Limitations of Relying on TSH Lab Testing Only 93

The Problems with T4-Only Therapy 94

Why Thyroid Conditions are So Commonly Missed 97

Chapter Highlights 99

How to Get Tested Correctly 101

Using Lab Tests to Determine Thyroid Function 101

Preparation For Testing 101

The Functional Approach to Thyroid Lab Testing 104

Thyroid Antibodies 106

Reverse T3 108

Thyroid Blood Test Panels 109

Thyroid Lab Patterns 111

Additional Labs Worth Considering 113

The Role of Thyroid Ultrasound 119

ThyroFlex Testing: 120

Chapter Highlights 122

Optimizing Thyroid Medications 123

An Introduction and Brief History of Thyroid Medication 123

Do You Need Thyroid Medication? 124

Which Medications Work Best? 125

Synthetic vs. Natural Desiccated Thyroid (NDT)? 127

Synthetic T4 Medication - Levothyroxine 128

Synthetic T4/T3 Medication 129

Synthetic T3 Medication 129

Slow-Release T3 131

Natural Desiccated Thyroid (T4/T3) 132

Controlling Fillers Compounded Thyroid Medication 134

Chapter Highlights 136

The Best Thyroid Diet 137

Core Principles of a Healthy Eating Plan 137

The Benefits of Organic Produce 143

Grains 145

Meat, Poultry, Fish, and Eggs 150

Sugar, Frankenfoods, and Other Proinflammatory Foods 153

Genetically Modified Foods, Pesticides, and The Thyroid........156

Is an Elimination Diet Right for You? 159

Autoimmune Paleo Diet 163

Chapter Highlights 164

Best Supplements for Thyroid Disorders................................165

Essential Nutrients for Optimal Thyroid Function.....................165

Nutritional Deficiencies 166

How to Identify Nutrient Needs....................................167

Making TSH & Supporting Pituitary Function.......................168

The Building Blocks of Thyroid Hormone..........................170

Important Autoimmune /Anti-Inflammatory Thyroid
Supplements......................................173

Improving Thyroid Hormone Conversion 177

Liver Detoxification...............................179

Thyroid Receptor-Activating Nutrients 181

Supplements for Adrenal Health 183

Chapter Highlights 189

Lifestyle Changes that Matter 191

Stress – The Destroyer of Health 191

Your Stress Inventory and Ways to Manage Stress.................193

Vitamin S – Sleep! 195

The Role of Sleep......................................196

Sleep Apnea and Hypothyroidism..................................196

Insomnia 197

The Importance of Exercise 201

Over-Exercise, Cortisol, and Thyroid Disorders..........202

The Paradox of Exercise and Low Thyroid.................203

Mindfulness and Emotional Restoration 205

Take Time for Yourself 207

Chapter Highlights...208

Taking Charge of Your Health................................209

Be Your Own Advocate...209

Where to Start 210

Ask Your Provider for Comprehensive Lab Tests........210

Getting Your Own Labs Done 211

Making Lifestyle Changes 211

Keep Learning!...213

Staying Objective/Develop a BS Detector! 213

Support Groups – Pros and Cons............................213

Good Online Resources...214

Finding a Practitioner Who Can Help 214

Functional Medicine Societies 215

Naturopathic Physicians.......................................215

How to Interview a Practitioner 216

Next Steps and Final Thoughts 217

Take Action 218

Learn More 218

Work with Me 219

Please Don't Keep Me a Secret! 219

Testing Resources 221

Standard Blood Testing Services 221

Specialty Labs 222

Reading List 225

Bibliography 227

This book is dedicated to my wife, Judith for her unconditional support, and to my daughter, Esperanza who did her best as a 5-year-old could to let daddy write. Yes, we can play Legos now. They have both been amazingly patient throughout this writing process.

I also want to dedicate this to all the thyroid patients seeking better health care options and I hope they find the answers to all their questions within this book.

Disclaimer

Free Bonus Videos

This book includes **free videos, cheat sheets**, and **guides** that help guide in your quest for better thyroid health.

To claim your free gifts, and learn more about how to improve thyroid function, go to the book website at:

www.thethyroidfixbook.com/bonus

Introduction

Why I Wrote This Book

IN MY NEARLY 20 YEARS OF CLINICAL PRACTICE, I've helped thousands of patients reverse their hypothyroid symptoms and rebalance their health. Much of this has been through educating my patients on lifestyle changes and convincing them to think about their thyroid condition holistically, which is essential for identifying and treating the root cause.

As I write this, the conventional medical wisdom of testing the thyroid with TSH alone and prescribing thyroid medication - typically a T4 replacement medication - is as common as it is misguided. This mechanistic approach has been long outdated. Unfortunately, the advancements in modern medicine are uneven. Some areas are remarkably cutting-edge, while other areas haven't changed in thirty years or more. This is especially true regarding the treatment of thyroid conditions.

As a result, many people with hypothyroid conditions are left to fend for themselves. Most are given levothyroxine (T4 replacement medication) and are told that any hypothyroid symptoms they are experiencing are related to something else entirely. For far too long hypothyroid conditions have either been left untreated or incorrectly diagnosed.

It is important to realize that much can be done to improve not just your hypothyroid symptoms, but your health overall. It is equally imperative to understand that many of these positive changes can be made by you, the reader, at home. This is what this book is all about. Self-advocacy is the guiding principle throughout every chapter. I believe it is essential that you take charge of your health.

Is This Book Right for You?

This book is written for people who have been diagnosed with hypothyroidism and experience symptoms associated with low thyroid function, such as fatigue, brain fog, poor memory, hair loss, hormone imbalances, and difficulty losing weight. If you can relate, then this book is for you!

Likewise, if you have been experiencing unexplained fatigue, weight gain, and problems with your hormones and have been told that your thyroid tests are normal and that you don't have a thyroid condition, then this book is for you too! Because most healthcare practitioners order only one test, they miss many low-functioning thyroid conditions that could be addressed using the approach outlined in this book.

To correct thyroid conditions I use a holistic, multi-system approach because the low functioning thyroid is a problem whose complexity extends well beyond the endocrine gland in the neck. It essential to look at the whole body and at times even outside the body to discover and treat the cause of thyroid conditions.

Most people experiencing low thyroid function are women, and as such, this book is primarily written with women in mind. However, men with hypothyroidism will benefit from this book as well. The guidelines found in the chapters apply equally to all genders.

If you are experiencing hyperthyroidism (Grave's disease), there are sections of the book that may offer benefit as well. That said, this book primarily addresses low functioning thyroid conditions such as hypothyroidism, Hashimoto's thyroiditis, thyroid hormone conversion disorders, and thyroid hormone receptor insensitivity.

The Holistic Approach to Thyroid Problems

The holistic or functional method takes a more logical and systematic approach to low functioning thyroid. There are many aspects of thyroid disorders that pertain to processes, conditions, and factors outside of the thyroid. If you are focused just on the thyroid – or like many conventional practitioners, only on the thyroid stimulating hormone (TSH) – then you miss many of the problems that cause the symptoms of low thyroid. Many practitioners simply dismiss these symptoms as relating to another condition because the symptoms fall outside their limited scope.

Many patients who are treated solely with T4-only thyroid replacement hormone are often left with low thyroid symptoms. Many of the patients who come to my clinic have been put on levothyroxine (T4) but haven't experienced the relief of symptoms that they expected. Again, this is because their former practitioner hadn't accounted for the thyroid as an entire system.

The Increasing Rates of Hashimoto's Thyroiditis

Hashimoto's thyroiditis, an autoimmune disease in which your white blood cells, called lymphocytes, attack your thyroid, has increased significantly in the past few decades. Conventional medicine has grossly mistreated this condition by merely providing thyroid hormone replacement which is increased over time as the overactive immune system eventually destroys the thyroid gland. The holistic approach to addressing the cause of Hashimoto's is outlined in this book as well.

Finally, and most importantly, hypothyroid conditions that are improperly addressed can have long-term consequences. Indeed, reduced quality of life is alarming enough, but the cardiovascular risk associated with the weight gain commonly seen with hypo-thyroidism is of particular concern. Moreover, Hashimoto's thyroiditis is associated with an increased risk of other autoimmune conditions, such as lupus and rheumatoid arthritis.

Ultimately, using this holistic approach not only helps reduce the symptoms and makes you feel better, but it also helps correct the course of thyroid disorders and moves you closer to optimal health. In some cases, there may not be a "cure" for a thyroid disorder, but with commitment and dedication to your health, you can feel so much better that you'll never allow yourself to go back to the way you felt before.

Who is Dr. Soszka?

Before we delve deeply into the world of thyroid health, I'd like to introduce myself. My name is Dr. Shawn Soszka. I'm a naturopathic physician and functional medicine practitioner with nearly 20 years of clinical experience working with thyroid patients. I have a busy functional medicine practice in Portland, Oregon with special focuses on thyroid and digestive disorders. In addition to a doctorate in naturopathic medicine, I also have a master's degree in oriental medicine and frequently use acupuncture and Chinese herbal medicine to treat thyroid conditions.

My Background

While I don't have a thyroid condition, I did suffer needlessly as a child from constant allergies and ear infections. I was so sick so frequently and so often in the pediatrician's office that the medical world became almost second nature to me. I was such a regular at the clinic that I received an anatomy coloring book from the clinic staff – and that was at age 3! As a child of the 70s, I probably spent more time on antibiotics than off. Over time, I developed allergies to the antibiotics, with a nearly fatal anaphylactic reaction to penicillin at age five. The cause of my constant ear infections turned out to be an undiagnosed milk allergy! My mother had her suspicions about milk but was repeatedly told that it couldn't possibly be the cause.

No doubt influenced by my health issues, I gravitated toward health care. However, due to the limited benefits I experienced with conventional medicine as a child, I developed a keen desire to find the root cause of a health condition and not just take symptoms at face value. It was this investigative mindset that led me to the comprehensive approach of naturopathic and functional medicine.

The Patient Who Changed the Course of My Career

Early in my career, I didn't have a specific health focus until I met a patient experiencing a severe form of Hashimoto's thyroiditis. At that time, I was working at one of the only integrative public health clinics in the area. One of the medical doctors that I worked with approached me with a patient's case and asked if I'd like to see her.

The MD expressed her frustration at not being able to help this patient, who was rapidly vacillating between severely low thyroid function to hyperactive thyroid function within a week's time. As such, the typical conventional medical approach didn't apply.

Through comprehensive thyroid testing, she was diagnosed with cyclical Hashimoto's thyroiditis. Now I admit, I couldn't help her back then as much as I could now, but my experience with her began my journey of learning as much as possible about treating the thyroid holistically.

Specializing in Holistic Thyroid Solutions

Since that time, I have had the privilege of meeting, getting to know, and learning from some of the thought leaders in the world of functional medicine and the holistic approach to thyroid conditions. I have had advanced training with Dr. Datis Kharrazian, Dr. Denis Wilson, and Dr. Daniel Kalish. I've also had the pleasure discussing the intricacies of Hashimoto's thyroiditis with Dr. Izabella Wentz, one of the most informed authorities on this subject.

I have been actively involved with promoting the holistic medical approach to thyroid and digestive disorders as a member of the Endocrinology Association of Naturopathic Physicians and as a founding board member of the Gastroenterology Association of Naturopathic Physicians. Additionally, I have served as adjunct professor at the National University of Natural Medicine, teaching functional gastroenterology to naturopathic medical students.

I hope you enjoy this book; there is a tremendous amount of information about thyroid conditions that people with low thyroid function never learn. I hope that this book helps you on your journey of healing.

Sincerely,

Dr. Shawn Soszka
Portland, Oregon, USA

CHAPTER 1

How the Thyroid Works

Thyroid: The Big Picture

THE FOCUS OF THIS BOOK IS THE THYROID GLAND, which is a small butterfly-shaped gland that sits between the Adam's apple and the base of the neck. It helps to have a basic understanding of how the thyroid works and of all the cells, tissues, and organs that thyroid hormone controls. The goal here is to give you a sense of the massive impact that the thyroid has on your overall health.

Thyroid hormones regulate the metabolism of every cell in your body apart from your red blood cells. Metabolism is the process of chemical reactions within cells to sustain life. This includes energy production, cellular repair and reproduction, and the specialized function of each of the different types of cells.

We're talking about brain and nerve cells, muscles, the digestive tract, reproductive organs, and so on. Specifically, thyroid hormone sets the speed at which cells operate and helps with the transformation of nutrients into energy within each of the cells.

For an example of how thyroid hormone affects the activity of a cell, let's take a look at the acid producing cells of the stomach. Normally, these cells produce stomach acid that helps break down food into smaller particles for easier absorption by the small intestines.

However, when the thyroid hormone is too low, these cells may only operate at 60% efficiency, producing far less stomach acid, not enough to break down food adequately. As a result, the nutrients from foods aren't absorbed well. By the way, this is a somewhat simplified summary. In the case of low thyroid hormone, all of the digestive tract would be affected, not just the stomach acid producing cells.

Thyroid hormones trigger the DNA in each of the cells to unravel small sections of the genetic code to produce proteins. These proteins help the cell do its job, be it a cell inside the eye that lets you see, or a cell lining the inside surface of the small intestine that helps with absorbing food. When these cells don't receive enough thyroid hormone, they work at a much slower pace and aren't able to perform all of their life-sustaining activities as efficiently.

The thyroid hormone also triggers the cells to produce energy in a specialized part of the cell called the mitochondria. The influence of thyroid hormone on energy production is massive because it controls, which is why fatigue is such a prominent symptom when there's not enough thyroid hormone.

Because of the massive impact that the thyroid has on the body, each of the steps in the process of creating, transporting, converting, and delivering the thyroid hormone to the cells needs to operate optimally for ideal health. When any step in the process is functioning poorly, the entire body can be thrown into chaos. For this reason, I think it's better to think of the thyroid as a system instead of merely as a hormone-producing gland.

To better understand the steps in the thyroid hormone system process, we will review this process step by step from the brain signaling to the delivery of the active thyroid hormone, T3, to the individual cell. I will also point out the differences between the functional and conventional medicine perspectives on thyroid function. Simply put, the main discrepancy is how each puts the science to use in a clinical setting. Functional medicine's approach to thyroid treatment uses the latest research, which informs patient care and treatment. I have encountered a lot of frustration from patients who felt that conventional medicine did not do enough in this regard.

It Starts in the Brain

Hypothalamus - The Master Regulator

The hypothalamus is a small, almond-sized part of the brain with a range of functions. For our purposes, however, it is important because it controls the endocrine system overall and produces a signaling hormone, thyroid releasing hormone (TRH), that is transported to the pituitary. The hypothalamus is key to creating a set point, like a thermostat, to regulate many systems in the body – blood pressure, body temperature, sex drive, and body weight, to name just a few.

The hypothalamus creates set points based on feedback from the amount of thyroid circulating in the body. If there is enough thyroid hormone in the bloodstream, the hypothalamus decreases the thyroid production signal. So far, so good. However, sometimes the feedback mechanism can become faulty, especially in the presence of inflammation. We will discuss this more in the next chapter.

Pituitary - The Master Endocrine Gland

The pituitary sits just below the hypothalamus and is often called the master gland as it controls the production of endocrine glands such as the thyroid, adrenal glands, testes/ovaries, and pancreas. While the pituitary may be the master gland, it takes orders from the hypothalamus, which sends thyroid releasing hormone (TRH) to the pituitary to adjust the output of its signaling hormone called Thyroid Stimulating Hormone (TSH) also called thyrotropin.

TSH is released from the pituitary and signals the thyroid to adjust the production of thyroid hormone. TSH is especially important to us because it is the primary lab measurement used in conventional medicine to track thyroid function. I will return to the topic of TSH lab testing repeatedly in this book because the current practice of using TSH as the only indicator of thyroid health is problematic. As with the hypothalamus, inflammation and other causes can reduce the responsiveness of the pituitary, which, in turn, can lead to low thyroid function.

The Thyroid

Remember that small butterfly-shaped gland sitting between the Adam's apple and the base of the neck? Yes, the thyroid, we've finally made it back. It is here that thyroid hormone is produced based upon the TSH hormone sent from the pituitary, which attaches to receptors on the thyroid and triggers thyroid hormone production. Once created, the thyroid releases the thyroid hormones into the bloodstream for delivery to the cells to regulate energy production and regulate metabolism.

Thyroid Hormone Production

I want to spend some time looking at how thyroid hormone is created. When TSH activates the thyroid, the thyroid jumps into action and actively increases its intake of iodine, a molecule that is essential for thyroid hormone production. This stimulates the creation of an enzyme called thyroid peroxidase (TPO) which helps attach iodine to thyroglobulin (TG), the molecule that thyroid hormone is created from. These are the fundamental building blocks of thyroid hormones, and they are subject to attack in thyroid autoimmune disease which is discussed in chapter 4.

The thyroid produces two hormones, a prohormone, Thyroxine (T4) and the hormone, Triiodothyronine (T3), both names based on the number of iodine molecules attached. Approximately 90% of the thyroid hormones produced are in the form of T4, with the remaining 10% produced as T3. The hormone T3 is the active form of thyroid hormone and is used by the different cells of the body. T4, on the other hand, has relatively little effect on the cells and must be converted to T3, which happens in the liver, intestines, muscles, brain, and kidneys.

How Thyroid Hormone is Transported

Once ready for release into the bloodstream, most of the thyroid hormones are chaperoned by the transport proteins, thyroid binding globulin (TBG), transthyretin, and albumin, with thyroid-binding globulin doing 90% of the work. When bound to these proteins the thyroid hormones are inactive and are carried to their destination tissue.

A small percentage of the thyroid hormones, T3 and T4, circulate freely in the bloodstream and can bind to the target cell and activate cellular production. A thyroid-binding globulin blood test can be useful when analyzing thyroid levels to determine any irregularities.

Thyroid Hormone Conversion

Because most circulating thyroid hormone is the less active T4, it must be converted into the active T3 for the body to make use of the hormone. This happens in several key locations, including the liver, intestines, kidneys, and, to a lesser extent, in the muscles and brain. Problems in any of these key locations can cause problems with thyroid hormone conversion.

This conversion of T4 into T3 occurs in the presence of an enzyme called *deiodinase* which removes one of the four iodine molecules from T4 hormone. Thus, the hormone becomes T3, named for the three remaining iodine molecules. Scientists have identified two rings on the thyroid hormone molecule that carries the iodine. They are referred to as the outer ring and the inner ring. This is important because when the iodine is removed the outer ring, the metabolically active T3 hormone is created. However, if the iodine is removed from the inner ring, the result is reverse T3 (rT3).

Reverse T3 is inactive but can still bind the thyroid hormone receptors at the cellular level. Not only is rT3 inactive, but it also inactivates all the receptors that it binds. Much like a key that fits a lock but doesn't open a door, reverse T3 prevents T3 from attaching to the blocked receptor. The net result is reduced metabolic activity. This is discussed in more detail in Chapter 3.

There are three subtypes of deiodinase enzymes aptly named Deiodinase 1 (D1), Deiodinase 2 (D2), and Deiodinase 3 (D3). These enzyme subtypes are found in different tissues of the body. While they all remove iodine from the thyroid hormones, they behave differently in different organs and enzyme activity can change depending on the overall health of the body.

Thyroid Hormone Receptors and Activation

Once converted, the T3 hormone is delivered to cells in all of the tissues in the body. It enters deep into the cell and attaches a T3 receptor at the nucleus to trigger protein production, one of the primary functions of cells. This is a vital part of cellular function because these proteins are fundamental to the operation of the cells.

As an example, the cone cells in the retina of the eyes allow us to see color. To do so, the cone cell produces a protein called opsin. When the T3 hormone attaches to the receptors of the cone cell, it triggers the production of opsin and, voilà, rainbows! Take this basic idea and multiply it by 30 trillion, the estimated number of cells in the human body. Because thyroid hormone affects every cell in the body (except red blood cells), thyroid disorders have the potential to be catastrophic to normal cellular function.

Another critical function of thyroid hormone is the regulation of energy production in the cells (called ATP) which is the source of all energy in the body. ATP is produced in the mitochondria, which serves as a power source for each of the cells. T3 hormone sets the rate by which the mitochondria operate. This is important because low functioning mitochondria produce less ATP, resulting in fatigue.

Chapter Highlights

- The thyroid has a massive impact on your body's function. Thyroid hormones regulate the metabolism of nearly every cell in your body. This includes energy production, cellular repair and reproduction, and the specialized function of each of the different types of cells.

- Because of the complexity and profound impact of thyroid hormone throughout the body, it is better to think of the thyroid as a system instead of merely as a hormone-producing gland. When any step in the process is functioning poorly, the entire body can be thrown into chaos.

- The hypothalamus and pituitary govern the production level in the thyroid by measuring the circulating thyroid hormone ensuring the body has adequate thyroid hormone to function properly.

- The thyroid primarily produces T4, which has limited activity in the body and must be converted to the biologically active, T3. This conversion occurs in several important organs including the liver, kidneys, and intestines.

- The T3 hormone is delivered to cells in all of the tissues in the body, triggering protein production and energy production.

CHAPTER 2

Do You Have Symptoms of Underactive Thyroid?

THERE ARE NEARLY 300 SYMPTOMS associated with low thyroid function. Undoubtedly, a considerable number of practitioners fail to associate many of these symptoms with the thyroid. In all fairness, the human body is very complicated and some of the symptoms listed below can occur because of other health conditions.

Recognizing the symptom patterns in thyroid dysfunction and confirming with the appropriate set of thyroid lab tests is key to making the correct diagnosis. Unfortunately, since most practitioners use only a single test to diagnose, many of these symptoms listed below are ignored or attributed to another cause.

Common Symptoms of Low Thyroid

The typical symptoms of hypothyroidism include the classic six symptoms: fatigue, goiter (throat and thyroid swelling), weight gain, cold extremities, hair loss, and constipation. These are some of the most obvious symptoms. Many other symptoms are either subtler or simply not associated with thyroid-related dysfunction among most healthcare practitioners.

The classic six symptoms present more commonly in moderate to severe hypothyroidism. Historically, hypothyroidism was caused by a lack of iodine in one's diet. For those who, for whatever reason, do not consume iodized salt today, this is still the case.

Because most people in the modern world who experience low thyroid symptoms are not suffering from the severe hypothyroidism seen in the past, their thyroid condition might get overlooked or misdiagnosed.

In recent decades, there has been a significant change in the cause of hypothyroidism. Growing at an alarming rate, autoimmune hypothyroid has overtaken iodine deficiency as the primary cause.

Throughout the book, I will be discussing thyroid dysfunction comprehensively, certainly in a way that transcends the narrowest definition of hypothyroidism. With that in mind, we will survey the other important causes of low thyroid function in the next few chapters.

Cognitive and Mood Symptoms

Brain and nerve cells depend on thyroid hormone to help generate energy and set the metabolic rate. Furthermore, research has found that the brain is saturated with thyroid hormone receptor sites where the thyroid hormone attaches and activates the cells. The fetal development of the brain depends on adequate thyroid hormone. Likewise, healthy brain function in adults is susceptible to thyroid hormone level changes. But it's a mutual relationship; the brain can influence thyroid function as well. We have two organs that work in conjunction and influence one another.

When thyroid hormone levels drop we begin to see signs of reduced brain function with cognitive symptoms such as short and long-term memory deficits, brain fog, poor concentration, and difficulty with basic computations. The brain produces neurotransmitters which are essentially the chemical of emotion. As thyroid hormone levels drop, these neurotransmitters drop accordingly. As a result, we see progressively worsening mood swings because the neurotransmitter deficiencies associated with depression and anxiety become more pronounced.

The thyroid influences neurotransmitter production and release in the brain, but two neurotransmitters in particular affect thyroid function directly. A brief introduction of these brain chemicals is helpful to illustrate the interplay between the brain and the thyroid.

Serotonin, the primary neurotransmitter associated with depression, can negatively affect the hypothalamus-pituitary-thyroid axis, interrupting the regulation of normal thyroid function. Reduced TSH production is commonly found with low serotonin. Furthermore, research indicates that those taking depression medications do not experience the maximum benefit from these medications until the underlying thyroid dysfunction is addressed.

Dopamine is commonly described as the "feel-good" neurotransmitter. This is why substances that raise dopamine levels such as caffeine, chocolate, and many recreational drugs are popular. As with serotonin, low dopamine levels reduce the effectiveness of the hypothalamus to regulate thyroid production. Low TSH levels are commonly the result. Additionally, dopamine plays an essential role in the conversion of T4 to T3 in the brain.

Both serotonin and dopamine are created from the amino acid, tyrosine, which is also one of the buildings blocks of thyroid hormone. While tyrosine deficiency is rare, because your body makes this amino acid, there are genetic conditions that prevent proper utilization of tyrosine.

Digestive Symptoms

Digestive symptoms often occur with thyroid disorders as the entire digestive tract from the mouth to the rectum moves slower and is less efficient. Constipation is one of the most common symptoms of low thyroid affecting the digestive tract. This has more impact than one might expect.

Nutritional deficiencies, such as iron, folate, zinc, calcium, vitamins A, D, and B12, are common among all those affected by low thyroid due to reduced stomach acid production. Low digestive enzyme production in the pancreas can compromise food absorption in the small intestine.

Likewise, low thyroid can increase the risk of intestinal infections and parasites! One digestive condition that I see commonly in my practice is small intestinal bacterial overgrowth (SIBO) which impedes nerve function and slows down movement in the small intestines. This can be caused by toxins produced by infectious bacteria, which paralyze the nerve cells. SIBO may also be triggered by low thyroid function which can bring the digestive tract to a virtual standstill!

Some other digestive symptoms of low thyroid include gas, bloating, abdominal tenderness or pain, hard stools, bad breath, reduced appetite, and the feeling of an overly full stomach.

Skin Symptoms

Since thyroid hormone influences skin cell growth and proper function, one hallmark of low thyroid function is dry skin. In addition to dryness, other skin-related symptoms of low thyroid include eczema, slower healing, bruising easily, and water retention in the deeper layers of the skin. It is also common to see weak and brittle fingernails and toenails.

Similarly, slower hair growth leads to hair thinning and often growing back coarser with a loss of the shine and luster of healthy hair. Finally, another hallmark of low thyroid function is the loss of the outer third of the eyebrows.

Musculoskeletal Symptoms

Another common symptom of low thyroid is increased muscle and joint pain. When there is not enough thyroid hormone, the muscle and joint cells are less active, and their ability to repair themselves is reduced.

Fibromyalgia is common among those with low thyroid function, especially those with either thyroid hormone resistance and/or autoimmune thyroid conditions, such as Hashimoto's thyroiditis.

If you have fibromyalgia, you should seriously consider comprehensive thyroid testing and evaluation. The thyroid isn't the only cause of fibromyalgia, but the connection is frequently overlooked.

Special Focus: Fatigue

Low energy is one of the most common complaints for which people seek medical attention. Feeling tired and having difficulty getting through the day makes life challenging. There are many causes of fatigue, so it is essential to investigate the nature of your symptoms. Documenting your symptoms in a fatigue journal may help a doctor determine the nature of your fatigue and discover its root cause.

One way a savvy healthcare practitioner can figure out the cause of fatigue is by asking important questions, such as: When are you most tired? Does activity worsen or improve fatigue? Does your fatigue worsen or improve throughout the day? Is your fatigue physical (such as muscle weakness), more cognitive (brain fog, poor memory), or both?

Keep in mind, a lack of nutrients usually causes fatigue. This can include oxygen and available thyroid hormone!

Let us look at some possible causes of fatigue and then compare them to low thyroid function.

IRON DEFICIENCY is a common cause of fatigue, but if this is the case, you will likely notice a pallor on tongue and fingernails. You'll also feel worse with exercise. Even climbing a flight of stairs may leave you out of breath due to a lack of available oxygen. Insomnia is also a common symptom of low iron; it is less common in low thyroid function. But some signs overlap; hair loss, for example, is shared with both iron deficiency and low thyroid. Low thyroid function can be a cause of iron deficiency, as it is nine times more common in those with low thyroid function than in those with normal thyroid function.

VITAMIN B12 DEFICIENCY is another relatively common medical condition that saps stamina. What's different than iron anemia is that the fatigue symptoms are mainly associated with poor memory and brain fog. Although these two symptoms are also common in low thyroid, B12 deficiency includes neurological symptoms, such as numbness and tingling in the arms and legs. More severe B12 anemias can lead to weakness of the limbs. I've seen patients who are so deficient that they had problems walking. In fact, one patient was bound to a wheelchair. With proper treatment, however, she was walking again in a month.

SLEEP APNEA is a condition in which the airway becomes blocked during sleep, reducing oxygen intake. It is common among overweight people. Now, most conventional healthcare practitioners are aware of the importance of screening for sleep apnea as the condition increases the risk of obesity, heart disease, and stroke. Keep in mind that sleep apnea may have its origins in low thyroid function, but for now let us consider the symptoms alone for the sake of comparison.

Typically, fatigue is at its worst when you first wake up and slowly improves during the day. More severe forms of sleep apnea reduce sleep quality to such an extent that one may feel tired all day. Other common symptoms of sleep apnea are nightmares, snoring, waking up choking, waking with a headache, and weight gain.

Now let's look at the fatigue symptoms of low thyroid function. I often see a combination of both physical fatigue – reduced endurance and muscle weakness – and what I call cognitive fatigue – brain fog, difficulty finding the right word, misplacing items, and short-term memory loss. Of course, I often find these along with the other common thyroid symptoms of cold intolerance, hair loss, constipation, and weight gain.

One of the interesting aspects of low thyroid-based fatigue is that it often improves with exercise temporarily. This occurs because activity increases metabolism and circulation, makes thyroid receptors more likely to accept thyroid hormone and can help with thyroid hormone conversion. One of the risks of exercise with low thyroid is over-exercising. What might be a good workout for a person in perfect health can worsen your thyroid condition. For this reason, I have included a special section in chapter 11 outlining effective exercise strategies for those with thyroid conditions.

Special Focus: Weight Loss

Weight gain and a struggle to lose weight are common in thyroid disorders. This is due to the lower metabolism, which conserves fat on the body as is the case of a bear in hibernation. As mentioned previously in chapter 1, one of the thyroid hormone's primary functions is to produce energy in the form of ATP in the mitochondria.

When thyroid hormone is insufficient or unable to enter cells, energy production will lag, and the body will interpret this as food scarcity. The body then goes into survival mode, reducing all bodily functions inessential to survival. From a survival perspective, having extra fat on the body is a positive attribute as it offers a reserve of nutrients, like a savings account that can be drawn upon in times of need.

Of course, most of those with thyroid conditions are not lacking in food; they lack in nutrients. It is essential to evaluate your nutritional status to determine if you are deficient in any of the critical vitamins or minerals that play a role in thyroid production, conversion, and cellular activation.

There is one exception to weight gain among thyroid conditions. In Hashimoto's thyroiditis, we may see average weight or even weight loss in the early stages of the disease. This is due to the destructive nature of this autoimmune disease, which releases stored pockets of thyroid hormone as the thyroid gland is destroyed by white blood cells. This results in symptoms of hyperthyroidism – which includes weight loss, or, at least, no weight gain – along with the more persistent symptoms of hypothyroidism, such as fatigue and hair loss.

Special Focus: Hormone Imbalance

Problems with the reproductive system are common with thyroid disorders, and imbalances between the sex hormones estrogen, progesterone, and testosterone can further compound the effects of low thyroid.

Most sex hormones are produced in the ovaries and testicles. Like the thyroid, the ovaries and testes are part of the endocrine system. As such, they are susceptible to imbalances of other endocrine glands because of the feedback loops that keep the system in balance.

The hypothalamus, first mentioned in the last chapter, regulates the sex hormones just as it controls the thyroid. The pituitary gland produces the signaling hormones that trigger production of the sex hormones. Problems arise if there is any dysfunction in either the hypothalamus or pituitary. This can range from a tumor in the pituitary to nutritional deficiencies and inflammation altering the functioning of these organs. Such complications can negatively impact production of the sex hormones.

As we have seen regarding other bodily functions, the decreased availability of thyroid hormone influences the production of the sex hormones. Among those with reduced thyroid function, we find low testosterone in men and imbalances in estrogen and progesterone in women.

POLYCYSTIC OVARIAN SYNDROME (PCOS) is a common condition among women ages 18 to 44 and is associated with elevated testosterone and other androgens (male hormones) that may cause male pattern body hair growth, acne, and irregular or absent menstrual cycles. Obesity is common with this condition. Likewise, low thyroid function, elevated blood sugar, and insulin resistance are widely seen.

Some scientists claim that low thyroid doesn't cause PCOS. Instead PCOS triggers hypothyroidism. Others argue that the thyroid, central to all body functions, is the key to addressing PCOS. I prefer taking into account all aspects of the condition: treating thyroid, regulating blood sugar, and normalizing hormones. The fundamentals of my approach can be helpful in addressing this condition.

INFERTILITY, defined as the inability to become pregnant after 12 months of consistent effort, is becoming more common today. It is estimated that one in ten women of childbearing age are affected. There is a very strong relationship between low thyroid function and infertility. The hormone T3 is essential for reproduction and a healthy pregnancy. In my practice, I've seen several cases of infertility resolved with the addition of a low dose of T3 medication. This is especially true for those with thyroid hormone conversion problems. Certainly, it is not the cure-all; it is necessary to look at all deficiencies that can either cause or be caused by low thyroid function. Ultimately, if fertility is an issue for you, it is worth looking closer at the thyroid.

MISCARRIAGE is an unfortunate reality most commonly associated with genetic defects that develop in the fetus resulting in miscarriage usually within the first trimester. By and large, this is more common in women with thyroid conditions as adequate thyroid hormone is necessary to ensure proper growth of the fetus. Looking at the levels of T3 thyroid hormone is very important in addressing the risk of miscarriage. Any woman with a history of miscarriage should be evaluated for low thyroid function and especially for Hashimoto's thyroiditis, which also increases the risk of miscarriage.

PREMENSTRUAL SYNDROME (PMS) is common in menstruating women and results in a variety of symptoms, most commonly water retention, back pain, breast tenderness, and mood fluctuations that typically begin 5 to 7 days before menses. This is most commonly associated with fatty acid deficiency, both omega-3, and omega-6, but women with thyroid disorders are more likely to experience PMS, and with more severe symptoms, than those with normal thyroid function.

Chapter Highlights

- Thyroid hormones drive the cellular metabolism of the body. Any thyroid hormone deficiency can reduce the normal function of the organs of the body. As a result, low thyroid function may manifest as a myriad of symptoms not classically associated with hypothyroidism.

- Insufficient thyroid hormones have a marked effect on cognitive function and mood. Low thyroid function may cause the onset of depression or anxiety.

- Digestive symptoms along with decreased nutrient absorption are common in low thyroid disorders. As a result, poor nutrition develops, further compounding the problem.

- Low energy is one of the most common complaints for which people seek medical attention. Because thyroid hormone drives energy production on a cellular level, it should always be considered when looking for the cause of low energy.

- Weight gain and a struggle to lose weight are common in thyroid disorders. This is due to the lower metabolism due to insufficient thyroid hormone.

- Additionally, the vitamin and mineral deficiencies common in thyroid disorders triggers the body to prevent weight as it enters survival mode during a period of perceived famine.

- Problems with the reproductive system are common with thyroid disorders, and imbalances between the sex hormones estrogen, progesterone, and testosterone can further compound the effects of low thyroid.

CHAPTER 3

The Many Causes of Low Thyroid Function

SO FAR, WE'VE REVIEWED HOW THE THYROID WORKS and the common symptoms of low thyroid function. Now we're going to dive deeper to explore the actual causes of low thyroid. There are many, so many, in fact, that I plan to expand upon several of this topic in upcoming books.

As I've mentioned before, the conventional medical world holds a rather static view on the thyroid. The consensus is that if the thyroid isn't meeting the body's demand for thyroid hormone, then it must be "broken" and that the patient needs the appropriate dosage of thyroid medication in the form of levothyroxine (T4) to make up for the deficit. Hypothyroidism is diagnosed, and treatment is monitored through the blood test thyroid stimulating hormone (TSH).

Unfortunately, this theory fails to address several critical aspects of thyroid disorders. First, both nutritional deficiencies and inflammation can negatively impact every aspect of the thyroid process. Additionally, when there are thyroid production problems associated with thyroid tissue destruction, most commonly occurring in the autoimmune condition, Hashimoto's thyroiditis, conventional medicine fails to offer any effective way of stopping the autoimmune process.

Furthermore, merely addressing thyroid conditions by replacing thyroid fails to address thyroid conditions that occur outside of the thyroid itself, including thyroid conversion disorders and thyroid hormone resistance at the cellular level. The thyroid, as a system, is far more complex than most conventional practitioners realize. Additionally, conventional medicine does not typically focus on nutrition as a therapy and therefore has little to offer besides thyroid medication mentioned above.

Signaling and Feedback Errors in the Brain

The hypothalamus tightly regulates thyroid hormone production. Continually monitoring thyroid hormone levels in the blood, the hypothalamus either increases or decreases the release of its signal to the pituitary, which, in turn, adjusts the production of TSH.

As previously mentioned, TSH is the pituitary hormone that controls the production of thyroid hormone. This process is meant to keep thyroid hormone at precisely the right level to keep the body operating normally. The interplay between these three glands is often called the Hypothalamus-Pituitary-Thyroid axis, often abbreviated as the HPT axis.

The assumption that the HPT axis functions normally, with the rare instance of damage to either the hypothalamus or pituitary, is one of the main reasons why conventional medicine only uses the TSH test. According to conventional (medical) wisdom, the thyroid gland itself is susceptible to damage due to autoimmune disease, and TSH accurately detects all abnormalities in the thyroid. But if this worked without fail, I wouldn't be writing this book.

However, the HPT axis is subject to dysfunction that can alter the accuracy of the esteemed TSH. This is yet another reason comprehensive thyroid testing is needed because we live in a time in which toxicity, inflammation, and nutritional deficiencies are more common than ever. All three of these factors can disrupt normal hypothalamus and pituitary function.

When looking for the cause of a thyroid disorder, it is common to start at the thyroid gland. This is a rational approach considering that autoimmune-induced hypothyroidism is so common. However, when the thyroid gland is intact and seemingly normal, but some aspect of the comprehensive thyroid lab results just isn't right, we must turn our attention to the regulators of the thyroid cycle, the hypothalamus, and pituitary.

Some diseases damage the structure of these two glands such as tumors, autoimmune diseases, brain injuries, and so on. The symptoms of such tissue damage are often dramatic and lead to significant health crises which are the domain of endocrinologists who are adept at diagnosing and treating such conditions.

For our purposes, I'd like to focus on the comparatively subtle impacts on the hypothalamus and pituitary glands such as chronic inflammation or nutritional deficiencies that disrupt the feedback mechanism. These situations can cause the feedback mechanism to incorrectly interpret the body's thyroid needs. As a result, the blood test so commonly used, TSH, will come back as either normal or even low, suggesting that the body is either getting enough or even too much thyroid hormone. In short, test results may fail to indicate what is occurring.

A number of studies have found chemicals called cytokines (especially IL-beta, IL-6, and TNF-alpha) are often elevated with inflammation which is associated with chronic stress, poor diet, and chronic illness. Likewise, elevated levels of cortisol, the adrenal stress hormone, are commonly found in these situations. All of these make the hypothalamus and pituitary less effective at keeping thyroid hormone at an optimal level because they impede production of the signaling hormones from the hypothalamus and pituitary (TRH and TSH, respectively).

The increase in inflammation greatly reduces the activity of the thyroid at all levels because the body associates high levels of inflammation with injury and illness. Normally, the body will reduce the metabolism allowing the body to rest and recuperate. However, this is no longer the only cause of inflammation. In our modern industrialized world, so many inflammation-causing agents enter our bodies in the form of foods, preservatives, colorings, pesticides, and other chemicals. As a result, someone may experience symptoms that are consistent with hypothyroidism but test normal for TSH.

There is plenty of research that demonstrates this process. Conventional medicine recognizes that the function of the hypothalamus and pituitary can be negatively affected, triggering either secondary or tertiary hypothyroidism. This is not difficult to diagnose if practitioners use the tests that provide the actual thyroid hormone levels in addition to TSH. Unfortunately, the TSH-only approach to diagnosis has become the "medical habit" of most practitioners as a cost-saving measure.

Likewise, inflammation can alter the normal function of the deiodinase enzymes responsible for converting T4 to the active T3. As previously mentioned, there are three deiodinase subtypes. Of the three, D2, is the most common type found in the hypothalamus and pituitary. This is important because the D2 subtype is less affected by inflammation than the two other subtypes, which are found in the liver and other tissues responsible for peripheral thyroid hormone conversion. So, the hypothalamus would likely indicate sufficient thyroid hormone in the bloodstream when the other tissues in the body don't have enough thyroid hormone to function properly.

Nutritional deficiencies can alter the normal function of the hypothalamus and pituitary. This is the case when you are deficient in key nutrients such as iron, vitamin A, zinc, chromium, and essential fatty acids. Such deficiencies reduce the ability of the hypothalamus to accurately detect circulating thyroid hormone or correctly produce the signaling hormone, TRH. As a result, thyroid production suffers due to the lack of feedback from the hypothalamus.

Since the hypothalamus regulates many functions in the body, it is common to see other symptoms not as commonly associated with low thyroid function such as poor temperature control and irregular blood pressure, especially with position changes (sitting to standing, etc.).

Nutrient deficiencies affect the pituitary in the same way and with the same results. TSH levels remain low or normal depending on the severity. The body's thyroid needs go unaddressed. When the pituitary isn't working correctly it is common to see problems with other endocrine glands in addition to thyroid symptoms. This can manifest in many ways – low cortisol due to decreased adrenal function, blood sugar irregularities associated with insulin production, and certainly sex hormone imbalances.

For instance, women are likely to experience menstrual irregularities and men lower testosterone levels. Admittedly, many of these symptoms are seen in low thyroid function. The savvy practitioner will not take the TSH lab results at face value but will investigate further.

Thyroid Hormone Conversion Disorders
Now let's take a look at low thyroid conditions that are not considered to fit the narrow medical definition of hypothyroidism, which, succinctly stated, is the inability of the thyroid to produce adequate thyroid hormone. That said, it is possible to have both hypothyroidism and a thyroid hormone conversion disorder.

At particular risk are those who have been prescribed synthetic T4 medication, levothyroxine, but have failed to experience an improvement in their thyroid symptoms. If you can relate, then read on. This chapter is written especially for you.

I find the conditions discussed below to be more common than hypothyroidism. Regrettably, they are very often ignored or attributed to another condition altogether, such as depression.

What is a Thyroid Hormone Conversion Disorder?

As mentioned earlier, about 80% of thyroid hormone produced by the thyroid gland is in the form of less active prohormone thyroxine (T4), which is then turned into the metabolically active triiodothyronine (T3) thyroid hormone. Most of the conversion process takes place in the liver and kidneys. The rest of the conversion occurs in the intestine and peripheral tissues.

Thyroid hormone conversion disorder is a condition in which the conversion process is either reduced to the point that T4 cannot convert into T3 or when T4 conversion is altered into creating the metabolically inactive Reverse T3 (rT3). These two aspects of the disorder lead to the same outcome: insufficient T3 thyroid hormone, resulting in symptoms of low thyroid function.

Several factors cause or contribute to thyroid hormone conversion disorder. Factors that we will consider include the body's toxic burden, nutrient deficiencies, imbalances between the adrenal glands and the thyroid, and liver and kidney disorders. We will look closely at liver, digestive, and adrenal dysfunction and how these relate to thyroid hormone conversion disorders and overall thyroid dysfunction in Chapter 4.

As discussed in Chapter 2, the deiodinase enzyme converts T4 into T3 by removing one of the four iodine molecules attached to the T4, creating T3. There are three subtypes of deiodinase enzymes, which the scientists cleverly named D1, D2, and D3. These enzymes are found all throughout the body, but more abundantly in certain tissues and organs. All of the deiodinase enzymes share the basic function of removing iodine, but each subtype does so in a different manner.

Deiodinase D1

The D1 enzyme, predominant in the liver and kidney, can re-move iodine from either the outer or inner rings and can therefore produce T3 or rT3. Research indicates that D1 enzyme activity is lower in women, making them more prone to thyroid disorders than men, especially low thyroid function when TSH levels are normal. In a moment we'll look at how D1 can be inhib-ited to create more reverse T3 than T3.

Deiodinase D2

The D2 enzyme is primarily found in the thyroid, heart, skeletal muscle, fat, hypothalamus, and pituitary tissues. Most importantly it is the only form of deiodinase enzyme found in the pituitary. It removes iodine from the outer ring only, meaning that it can only make the active T3 molecule from T4. It also breaks down re-verse T3 into T2 which is an inactive thyroid molecule that has two iodine molecules.

The D2 enzyme, found deep within the cell, plays an important role in ensuring there is enough T3 in the normally functioning cell. Since D2 is the only form of deiodinase in the pituitary, TSH, TSH may not reflect a T4 conversion disorder in the other tissues such as the liver or kidneys. In situations such as inflammation, chronic illness, or pain, the D1 enzyme will con-vert more T4 to reverse T3 than desired. Because the pituitary can only produce T3 and not rT3, the TSH produced in the pitui-tary may look normal when the body needs more thyroid hor-mone.

Deiodinase D3

The D3 enzyme, found in all tissues of the body except the pituitary, and most plentifully in fetal tissue and the placenta, plays an important role in the healthy development of the fetus during pregnancy. D3 removes iodine from the inner ring only and, thus, produces reverse T3 only.

D3 plays an important role in preventing overexposure of T3 in the cell. The deiodinase system controls the amount of T3 within the cells and serves as the regulator of the cellular activity of intracellular thyroid hormone. It also helps to free iodine for other uses inside the cell. When functioning properly, it keeps thyroid hormone levels in balance. However, situations such as nutrient deficiencies, cortisol imbalance, inflammation, severe calorie restriction, low-carb diets, and certain medications can alter the normal function of these enzymes, resulting in reduced conversion or shifts toward reverse T3. In Chapter 8 I will explain in greater detail why a low carbohydrate diet is a bad idea for those with low thyroid function.

Decreased Thyroid Hormone Conversion

As described in the previous section, three deiodinase enzymes are responsible for the conversion of thyroid hormones. Each of these enzymes converts thyroid hormone differently in different tissues of the body. We will now look at several factors that influence the conversion process. There are enough factors to warrant a separate book on the subject, one I intend to write.

External factors also influence these enzymes, each in a different way. As an example, the D1 enzyme – again most commonly found in the liver and kidneys – is highly susceptible to the effects of environmental pollution. Thus, exposure to pesticides and pollutants decreases the conversion of T4 to T3. These environmental toxins do not appear to affect the D2 enzyme, primarily found in the pituitary. Even when the D2 is exposed to toxins, T4 to T3 conversion and TSH levels are normal. The net result:

low thyroid symptoms without indication of anything abnormal, at least, based on the conventional medicine model of thyroid testing.

Nutritional Deficiency

Poor nutritional status is another factor of poor thyroid hormone conversion. In this respect, the two minerals that stand out are selenium and iron. While selenium plays an essential role in thyroid hormone production within the thyroid gland, it is also a critical nutrient in the thyroid hormone conversion process in the form of selenocysteine.

This protein, a combination of the amino acid cysteine and selenium, is vital for the formation of the three deiodinase enzymes. A deficiency of this protein dramatically hinders the conversion process. Selenium supplementation is only a part of the solution. You will also need other nutrients involved in the thyroid hormone conversion process, such as zinc, B vitamins (especially B6 and B12), and magnesium.

Similarly, iron deficiency reduces the ability to convert T4 to T3 and further slows down metabolism, needed in so many of the chemical pathways of the body. Of course, low thyroid function will limit the ability to absorb iron, resulting in a vicious cycle. Due to poor absorption, common iron sources in your diet may not be enough to meet the demands of your body. Iron supplementation is likely needed until the thyroid hormone conversion disorder is either resolved or managed using T3 hormone replacement medication, such as Cytomel or the generic, liothyronine.

Genetics

Mutations in the DIO2 gene result in reduced deiodinase enzyme production or reduced effectiveness of the deiodinase enzymes. The DIO2 gene is responsible for the synthesis of the deiodinase enzyme. Heterozygous mutations, that is, one of the two pairs of genes being affected, result in mild to moderate impairment of deiodinase function. Homozygous mutation, in which both pairs of genes are mutated, causes more severe forms of thyroid hormone conversion impairment. Keep in mind that genetic testing shows a predisposition to impaired function, but doesn't necessarily indicate that function is, in fact, currently impaired.

DIO2 gene testing is commercially available. Until mid-2017, the popular genetic testing service, 23andme, tested at least one of the three sites of mutation found in the DIO2 gene. In late 2017, 23andme significantly reduced the number of genes tested, limiting its usefulness for clinical practice. I am currently working with a gene-testing company that promises to test more genes, including the DIO2 gene, in the near future. I will update this section once this test is available.

Reverse T3

As mentioned earlier in this chapter, reverse T3 is the metabolic inactive form of T3. It attaches to thyroid receptors, preventing an increase in cellular activity. Normally some amount of rT3 is produced during the thyroid hormone conversion process as a preventative for the overproduction of T3. In cases of chronic stress and inflammation, however, the different deiodinase enzymes shift toward less T3 conversion and more reverse T3 production. Additionally, it is common for individuals with high cortisol levels to show higher levels of rT3 as well, which results in symptoms of fatigue and stubborn weight gain. Many in this situation will gain weight with exercise!

It is also possible to experience the effects of high reverse T3 without having elevated rT3 detected in your labs. This occurs when T3 levels are low, but reverse T3 is in the normal range. The discrepancy results in low thyroid symptoms. I find this especially common in women who are experiencing higher levels of stress and inflammation and happen to have genetic variants to the DIO2 gene.

In addressing reverse T3 problems, the priority is to determine the blood levels of T3 and reverse T3. Some insist on looking at a lab called Free T3 (FT3) and comparing the amount of T3 hormone unbound to a carrier protein with the amount of reverse T3. Others prefer to look at the total T3 (TT3) and reverse T3. I check all three and look at the relative ratios of FT3/rT3 and TT3/rT3. If you are unfamiliar with these labs, I go into quite a bit of detail in chapter 7 about the best labs for assessing thyroid function and what the results reveal.

The second most important thing to do is to look at cortisol levels. Cortisol, produced by the adrenal glands, is often described as the "stress hormone" of the body. Stress drives up the production of cortisol to help reduce inflammation. As mentioned above, elevated cortisol shifts thyroid hormone conversion toward higher levels of reverse T3 and reduced T3 production. This is a natural response in the body, much like slamming on the brakes in your car to prevent a collision. I commonly recommend a saliva adrenal stress test to determine cortisol levels. This, along with a comprehensive thyroid panel, provides enough detail to address most thyroid hormone conversion issues.

Thyroid Hormone Resistance and Receptor Defects

Of the topics least discussed in most clinical settings is that of Thyroid Hormone Resistance, also known as Impaired Sensitivity to Thyroid Hormone (ISTH). For this section, we will use the latter term because it is more up-to-date. ISTH represents a class of conditions in which the thyroid receptors of individual cells cannot function properly.

In ISTH, T3 reaches the cells but cannot correctly bind to the defective receptor. This results in symptoms of low thyroid function, but without any of the thyroid hormone production issues associated with hypothyroidism.

There are several theories as to why this happens. Genetics appear to play a significant role in ISTH. A very well-written book by Hugh Hamilton, *Impaired Sensitive to Thyroid Hormone*, delves deeply into this topic. Initially, a genetic variation in the thyroid hormone receptor beta gene was associated with ISTH. The beta receptor gene mutation is rare, affecting 1 in 50,000.

Recent research, however, has found a similar genetic variant in the thyroid hormone receptor alpha gene, resulting in a similar thyroid hormone resistance. There are likely other genes with defects involved in thyroid hormone receptor production that have not yet been identified. Likewise, poor health, such as nutritional deficiencies and inflammation, can alter normal gene expression, reducing or impairing T3 receptors.

ISTH is not commonly known in the medical community and is often misdiagnosed as hyperthyroidism or as non-thyroid related fatigue. What's particularly insidious about ISTH is that those with all the symptoms of low thyroid function may have labs that come back normal.

In other ISTH cases, TSH may be normal or even high, T4 may be normal, and T3 may be high, but the symptoms of hyperthyroidism (weight loss, rate heart rate, sweating, anxiety) will be missing. In fact, a person with ISTH will likely have common hypothyroid symptoms (fatigue, difficulty losing weight, slow digestion, fibromyalgia-like aches and pains, and hormonal problems).

Additional factors that can impair the function of thyroid hormone receptors are abnormal cortisol and low iron levels. Those who have adrenal gland problems, such as adrenal insufficiency or adrenal fatigue syndrome, will have lower cortisol levels.

Adrenal insufficiency is more severe and occurs when the adrenal glands do not make enough cortisol, due to an autoimmune disorder called Addison's disease.

Adrenal fatigue syndrome is a less severe subclinical condition in which cortisol levels may be high or low, or the 24-hour cortisol rhythm is dysfunctional. In cases of thyroid hormone resistance, cortisol levels tend to be too low, which impairs the thyroid receptor function. Low iron levels have a similar effect, slowing down thyroid hormone receptors. Please see chapter 5 to learn more about the role of the adrenal glands on low thyroid function and chapter 9 to learn more about optimal iron levels.

Chapter Highlights

- Inflammation and nutritional deficiencies can disrupt the normal function of the hypothalamus and pituitary resulting reduced responsiveness to low circulating thyroid hormone levels.

- The conversion of T4 to T3 can be negatively impacted by inflammation, nutrient deficiency, stress, and dysfunction of the major organs involved in the conversion process. This results in low thyroid function independent of thyroid production.

- Excess reverse T3 disables thyroid hormone receptors within the cells resulting in reduced metabolic function and energy production.

- Thyroid hormone resistance occurs when the thyroid hormone receptors within the cells of the body do not function normally due to genetic, nutritional, or inflammatory factors.

CHAPTER 4

Hashimoto's Thyroiditis

HASHIMOTO'S THYROID DISEASE deserves a chapter unto itself since it is the most common form of hypothyroid condition in the industrialized world and is only increasing in frequency, affecting individuals younger than ever before.

Hashimoto's is an autoimmune condition in which the body's immune system mistakenly identifies proteins within the thyroid as foreign material and attacks thyroid tissue, which over time is replaced by scar tissue. The thyroid is capable of regenerating itself, but if too much scar tissue builds up, there is no chance of restoring the thyroid to normal function. When this occurs, permanent thyroid medication is needed.

As females are seven times more likely to develop Hashimoto's thyroiditis than males, it was previously thought that the condition was primarily caused by significant hormone fluctuations associated with puberty, postpartum, and menopause. While hormones can play a role in the development of Hashimoto's in women, science has found that among those with this condition a genetic predisposition is triggered by many factors, in addition to hormones.

This condition is especially worrisome because there is a risk of developing other autoimmune diseases and even thyroid cancer. The limited treatment options available in conventional medical practice leave those with Hashimoto's few solutions.

If you have been identified as hypothyroid, then chances are that you have Hashimoto's thyroiditis. You need to understand that there are numerous treatment methods that, by finding and addressing the underlying cause, can help, not just with treating the symptoms, but also with reducing the damage caused by the autoimmune process, which can save your thyroid.

Why Autoimmunity Goes Untreated

There is a misconception that autoimmune conditions, such as Hashimoto's thyroiditis, are untreatable. This is only true when you apply the conventional medical model, which merely treats symptoms by suppressing a chemical process or replacing a missing hormone (e.g., thyroid hormone or insulin).

The idea of making the body stronger and more resilient is a relatively new concept in conventional medicine that has not been adopted into clinical practice. I attribute this neglect to the surgical and drug origins of modern medicine which are based on treating life-threatening conditions.

Symptoms of Hashimoto's thyroiditis often occur after the autoimmune process has been active for at least a year, usually longer. The immune system attacks and destroys the thyroid cells. For thyroid hormone production to drop off to such an extent that it would trigger the classic hypothyroid symptoms would indicate that a significant part of the thyroid has already been damaged.

Because most practitioners don't screen for thyroid antibodies, the condition is only diagnosed after hypothyroidism presents. Keep in mind that the autoimmune attack occurs first and that hypothyroidism occurs after the disease has progressed significantly.

Much of the focus of this chapter is on increasing your awareness of this condition. I also provide lifestyle tools that you can use to feel better, and I address the autoimmune component as well. As mentioned before, you can start making these lifestyle changes at home, but I recommend working with a holistic practitioner who is "thyroid literate" for guidance through this process.

T4 Medication Doesn't Stop Thyroid Destruction

I think it is important to emphasize that thyroid hormone replacement medication given for hypothyroidism does nothing to address the autoimmune process. Many patients who have come to my clinic have been told that thyroid medication will help with their Hashimoto's hypothyroidism. They get quite upset when they find out later that nothing has been done to reduce the thyroid antibodies which have been destroying the thyroid cells all along.

Since thyroid hormone replacement medication is the only therapy that is offered in conventional medical settings, the autoimmune process persists, and the antibodies continue to destroy the thyroid gland and replace it with scar tissue. Essentially, most practitioners wait for the thyroid to die off so that a stable dose of thyroid medication – typically levothyroxine (T4) – can be prescribed.

The holistic medical practitioner has many more tools available to help address the autoimmune process.

Your Thyroid is Under Attack!

Many factors trigger the white blood cells to attack the thyroid tissues. As we review the different causes of the autoimmune process, I recommend thinking back on your personal health history to see if you can relate to any of the triggers listed below.

In my clinical experience, I find that most Hashimoto's patients have a family history of thyroid disease. Even if they are not diagnosed, the symptoms of their family members will, at least, suggest some form of thyroid disorder. Sometimes the cause of Hashimoto's isn't apparent and additional testing is needed to uncover the trigger. We will discuss possible causes in detail in Chapter 5.

The thyroid gland is especially susceptible to damage due to the way it makes thyroid hormone. The use of hydrogen peroxide in the creation of thyroxine (T4) leads to a buildup of free radical oxygen molecules. Free radicals are molecular byproducts of cellular activity missing an electron, which they try to steal from other molecules in the cell. If allowed to build up, they become toxic to the cell. This buildup is called oxidative stress.

Naturally, the body has a mechanism to neutralize free radical buildup, but it requires adequate amounts of glutathione. Glutathione requires selenium as a key ingredient in its creation. It also needs vitamin C for proper function. I find that most patients with thyroid problems are lacking in both nutrients.

It is vitally important to address the autoimmune process because 1) it will eventually destroy the thyroid, and 2) this autoimmune process can spread to other parts of the body. In the pancreas, it causes autoimmune diabetes. In the joints, rheumatoid arthritis. In the skin, vitiligo, a disease in which the white blood cells kill the melanocytes responsible for skin color, resulting in patches of white, unprotected skin and an increased risk of skin cancer.

Now you understand the massive repercussions of Hashimoto's thyroiditis. The fact that conventional medicine does not address it other than to provide thyroid hormone replacement and if deemed necessary, to surgically remove the thyroid gland is a profound injustice to those individuals with this disease. This is one of the reasons why so many are looking for answers. Thankfully, much can be done to address this condition as we will discuss here and in later chapters of this book.

Genetics and Family History

Since research indicates a significant family history of thyroid conditions (either hypo- or hyperthyroid) among those with Hashimoto's thyroiditis, it is important to investigate your family history. We know that this condition is more common in women. Furthermore, several genetic markers have been identified as making a person more prone to autoimmune thyroid conditions.

Among the most common are the HLA-DR and CTLA4 genes. In my practice, I commonly find alterations to these genes among my Hashimoto thyroiditis patients. Like the DIO2 gene discussed in chapter 3, the 23andme.com genetic test profile (version 4) included these two genes until August 2017. Currently, the CTLA4 is still on the version 4 profile, but the HLA-DR gene variants have been significantly reduced, making the 23andme test far less helpful. Both of these genes are associated with increased risks of other autoimmune diseases, not only Hashimoto's thyroiditis.

That said, your genes do not determine your destiny. There is always a trigger that sets any autoimmune process in motion. Since genetics only governs predisposition, much like a fuse, which is harmless until lit, we must look at other factors to identify the flame that ignites the process.

The Causes of Hashimoto's Thyroiditis

Epstein-Barr Virus and Other Viral Causes

Epstein-Barr (EBV) is the virus that causes mononucleosis, also known as the "kissing disease." EBV is a member of the herpes family, designated as Human Herpesvirus 4. It is very common to have had an EBV infection in your lifetime. When tested, most people will show antibodies of a previous infection.

Historically, most people were exposed to EBV by age two and had symptoms so mild that an EBV infection was mistaken for a common cold. However, with better sanitation and hygiene practices, we are observing exposure occurring later in life with more severe symptoms: extreme fatigue, sore throat, swollen tonsils, etc. This usually lasts two to six weeks, more so for those who are infected in their 20s.

Most commonly, the immune system will fight the EBV virus until the virus goes dormant. Some will experience reactivation of EBV, which can trigger an autoimmune response in different tissues in the body, including the thyroid gland. Other viruses can act as triggers, including cytomegalovirus (CMV) and the far rarer Human herpesvirus 6 (HHV 6).

Intestinal Infections

For another potential cause of autoimmunity, we must turn our attention to the intestines. The large intestine is a favorable environment for bacteria, which is collectively called the microbiome. We have developed a symbiotic relationship with these bacteria. Unfortunately, there is a class of bacteria that is known to trigger autoimmune conditions, including Hashimoto's thyroiditis. In patients tested at my clinic, I have found intestinal infections that did not have any digestive symptoms. Eliminating these infections improved the Hashimoto's thyroiditis in these patients.

Yet another potential cause of autoimmunity is a condition commonly known as leaky gut, or intestinal permeability in medical circles. In leaky gut, gaps form between the cells lining the small intestine whose job is to break down and absorb nutrients. Once these gaps have formed, food particles, yeast, bacteria, and other microbes enter deep into the tissues where the intestinal immune system is located, which triggers inflammation and a strong immune response. The end results are reduced absorption and the body mistaking food for dangerous microbes. A strong immune reaction follows. I go into far more detail about this in chapter 5.

Hormonal Changes

Research indicates that common onset of Hashimoto's thyroiditis occurs at times of extreme hormonal fluctuations, such as puberty, childbirth, and menopause. A relatively new hormonal trigger is oral birth control. While the availability of birth control has been revolutionary for women, like any other medication, it is not without its downside. There has been significant research on the topic, and it appears that women with genetic disposition are more likely to develop autoimmune thyroid with the use of the oral birth control pills. Other forms of birth control do not appear to be problematic.

Toxins and Toxic Metals

Pollution is an unpleasant aspect of our modern age. There is plenty of research that indicates that pollutants like mercury and chemicals from plastics and other sources are potential triggers for Hashimoto's thyroiditis.

Other types of thyroid problems can occur due to toxins in the body. These include thyroid hormone conversion dysfunction, reduced thyroid hormone production, and increased thyroid hormone resistance at the cellular level. In all of these examples, toxins can reduce the absorption of nutrients and worsen inflammation. Certainly, thyroid hormone conversion tissues, especially the liver and thyroid hormone receptors throughout the body, can be negatively impacted by toxins, such as synthetic pesticides, chemicals used in plastics, heavy metals, and flame retardants.

While we all have some level of toxicity in our bodies, what matters most is how the body reacts to these toxins. This is often determined by the levels of antioxidants in the body, especially glutathione. When antioxidants, especially glutathione, are low, your body cannot manage the damage that toxins cause. If the toxins build up enough, your body may start producing antibodies to these substances, and you are far more likely to experience autoimmunity in your body, including your thyroid.

Radiation Exposure

In my clinical experience, I've seen several patients with a history of exposure to radiation. In one case, a woman in her sixties being treated for Hashimoto's thyroiditis had a history of significant dental issues and had undergone many x-rays of her mouth and neck. Unfortunately, she had not been provided with any sort of radiation protection, and as we began treatment, a thyroid ultrasound found a suspicious thyroid nodule and enlarged lymph node. Additional testing found that she had developed thyroid cancer, which had spread to nearby lymph nodes. Removal of the thyroid and affected lymph nodes was performed. As this case illustrates, Hashimoto's increases the risk of thyroid cancer. Whenever I see thyroid antibodies, I recommend thyroid ultrasound.

This is an excellent example of why I am keen on using thyroid ultrasound imaging as a screening tool and why current medical guidelines recommend it if thyroid nodules are found. I would even recommend a preliminary ultrasound for any person with elevated thyroid antibodies. I discuss this in depth in Chapter 6 when reviewing the best tests for thyroid.

The Symptoms of Hashimoto's Thyroiditis

The symptoms of Hashimoto's thyroiditis depend on how long the condition has been active. At first, most won't experience any significant symptoms. As the immune system continues its attack, we may see a mix of hyper- and hypothyroid symptoms that can present simultaneously.

As an example, classic hypothyroid symptoms of cold intolerance and fatigue may coexist with hyperthyroid symptoms, such as anxiety and palpitations. Since both Graves' disease (hyperthyroidism) and Hashimoto's thyroiditis are autoimmune conditions, some cases of Hashimoto's in a hyperthyroid state are misdiagnosed as Graves' disease. As the hyperthyroid phase shifts back into hypothyroidism, we see more symptoms of hypothyroidism.

Generally, hypothyroid symptoms are more common overall, with brief episodes of hyperthyroidism. This occurs because the attacking white blood cells destroy part of the thyroid containing pockets of stored thyroid hormone, which are then released into the bloodstream without any transport proteins attached. This causes the thyroid hormone to attach to nearby cells triggering increased metabolism in these areas only. Since the thyroid is located in the lower neck, the brain and heart may be affected. Increased activity may include rapid heart rate and anxiety. This is especially true in the early to mid-stages of the disease.

Weight issues are complicated in Hashimoto's thyroiditis as weight gain is a common symptom of hypothyroidism, but some individuals don't experience any weight gain. This lack of weight gain is especially true in those who test low for low salivary cortisol. In fact, I see weight loss as a symptom in about 30% of my Hashimoto's patients with deficient cortisol levels. Because weight gain is so ingrained in the minds of many practitioners, they often overlook the thyroid as the culprit of their patient's symptoms. Unfortunately, this delay in correct diagnosis allows the disease to progress even further, which perpetuates suffering.

Special Topics in Hashimoto's Thyroiditis

While discussing the intricacies of autoimmune thyroid disease, I want to bring to your attention two topics that are important for the recovery process for anyone with Hashimoto's thyroiditis.

In the first section, we will review the ongoing debate about iodine supplementation among the functional medicine community. I bring this up because you find differing opinions on the topic and I wanted to provide some background to enhance your understanding.

The second section is focused on low-dose naltrexone (LDN), often described as a wonder-drug because it has helped thousands to manage their autoimmune conditions. I've prescribed LDN to many of patients, and I share some the results I've seen with this medication.

The Iodine Controversy

I've named this section the "iodine controversy" because iodine has largely been ignored or vilified by the medical community. By "ignored," I mean that the current medical thinking has overlooked the effects associated with decreased intake of this vital nutrient. While "vilified" is perhaps a strong word, complete avoidance of iodine is often recommended by both the conventional and holistic medical communities for those with autoimmune thyroid conditions. I disagree with this approach.

We need iodine as it is a nutrient essential for thyroid hormone production. Furthermore, it plays an essential role in breast tissue health, has anti-cancer properties, and is critical for healthy fetal development during pregnancy. Additionally, iodine is well known for minimizing radiation damage.

The value of iodine is without question, but are we getting enough in our diet? Is there anything that might be blocking its absorption? Should it be avoided when you have autoimmune thyroid disease? Let's focus on answering each of these questions so that you can navigate the often confusing and contradictory information regarding iodine and thyroid disorders.

A Growing Deficiency?

Iodine deficiency has long been known as a cause of hypothyroidism, which was thought to be resolved when iodine was added to flour and salt in the 1920s. Iodization did appear to help prevent hypothyroidism considerably, and there may have even been the "side benefit" of raising the average IQ to a moderate degree. In the 1970s, in response to concerns about American getting too much iodine, it was replaced by bromine in the commercial flours in the U.S. Unfortunately, bromine suppresses thyroid function and can be toxic at high levels.

Since then, in most of the developed world, the primary source of iodine intake is through salt, which we are told to restrict due to concerns about the high blood pressure risk of sodium. In fact, 50% of our modern diet consists of processed foods that use non-iodized salt, resulting in excess sodium and insufficient iodine intake. You can still get iodine from foods, however, and I encourage you to do so using the list provided below. Those who eat seafood, and especially seaweed, tend to get enough iodine so sushi fans can rejoice.

Calling our attention back to salt, many people have gotten wise to the chemicals used for commercial table salt. As a result, many health-conscious individuals have switched to either sea salts or Himalayan salts because they contain trace minerals, including iodine. However, these salts only have small and inconsistent amounts of iodine.

Are we getting enough iodine from our soil? The answer is no. Iodine soil levels are deficient in many parts of the Midwest in the U.S. and Canada, though they are high in the coastal regions. Modern farming practices often deplete this mineral even in soils that are historically iodine-rich.

Supplementing with iodine in a multivitamin or a thyroid-specific vitamin formulation can be helpful, but I recommend performing an iodine urine test before taking any amount over 50 mcg. See chapter 7 to learn more about iodine testing.

Hashimoto's Thyroiditis and Iodine

In the holistic and functional medicine community, some practitioners adamantly oppose any iodine intake for those with autoimmune thyroid conditions, such as Hashimoto's thyroiditis or Graves' disease.

The rationale for this argument is that an increased intake of iodine, a key ingredient for making thyroid hormone, increases the production of the thyroid enzyme, thyroid peroxidase (TPO), which attaches iodine to the protein backbone that produces thyroid hormone. The increase in TPO enzyme triggers an increase in TPO antibodies, which makes the autoimmune thyroid condition worse. This argument's chief proponent is Dr. Datis Kharrazian, who strongly recommends avoiding iodine supplements and foods high in iodine, such as seaweed.

There are competing views, however. Dr. David Brownstein, a strong iodine advocate, argues that iodine deficiency remains a significant issue that is getting worse. He believes that among most of those with thyroid disorders, iodine deficiency either causes or contributes to their problems. Dr. Brownstein's research suggests that iodine deficiency may be a trigger for autoimmune thyroid conditions. As such, he believes that iodine use can be beneficial for all, including those with autoimmune thyroiditis. Dr. Brownstein recommends high doses of iodine for all cases of hypothyroidism.

I have found that none of my patients' thyroid antibodies have worsened when they supplement with iodine. Nevertheless, it is essential to balance iodine and selenium, as the latter helps reduce inflammation in the thyroid, and therefore, lowers antibody levels.

Low-Dose Naltrexone

First introduced in the 1970s, the medication Naltrexone is used as a treatment for alcoholism and opioid abuse at 100 mg. At this dosage naltrexone works by blocking opioid receptors where these substances would normally attach, thus preventing the "high" experienced by those who consume alcohol or opioids.

Shortly after Naltrexone was introduced, Dr. Bernard Bihari began prescribing very small doses, between 1 to 4.5 mg daily, to successfully treat many autoimmune conditions, cancer, and HIV/AIDS. It was from his work that the term "low-dose naltrexone," or "LDN," became known. When given below 4.5 mg, naltrexone partially blocks the receptors for a short time. This tricks the brain into thinking that levels are too low, and triggers increased endorphin production.

Individuals with autoimmune conditions typically have lower endorphin levels than their healthy counterparts. It's a bit of a mystery as to why endorphins work to help normalize the immune system and reduce inflammation. Ongoing research is trying to figure it out. I've used LDN for several years in my practice and have seen the most dramatic results in inflammatory bowel diseases, such as ulcerative colitis and Crohn's disease. The results are more mixed with Hashimoto's thyroiditis patients; I've had many cases with a significant drop in thyroid antibodies and others with no noticeable change.

The recommended approach for LDN dosage for Hashimoto's is to start lower: 1.5 mg for two weeks. Here's the rationale: a sudden drop in thyroid antibodies would likely kick-start the thyroid and reduce the need for medication. The caveat here is that this may induce a temporary hyperthyroidism if one doesn't adjust thyroid medication dosage accordingly. So, it's best to start slow and low. Here's the schedule I use for my Hashimoto's thyroiditis patients: 1.5 mg for the first two weeks, 3.0 mg for the next two weeks, and then 4.5 mg thereafter.

The use of LDN is technically "off-label," meaning that the FDA has not approved naltrexone for such use. Therefore, you need a compounding pharmacy to fill your prescription. (See the

Resources section for more information about finding a compounding pharmacist.) Side effects are minimal. You may experience poor sleep and vivid dreams the first two weeks of use.

Low-dose naltrexone is a very safe medication that has helped many people who had otherwise lost hope. Admittedly, the results experienced with LDN have been mixed in treating Hashimoto's thyroiditis, but it is still worth considering. LDN has been especially helpful for those with fibromyalgia and rheumatoid arthritis.

Chapter Highlights

- Hashimoto's thyroiditis is the most common form of hypothyroid condition in the industrialized world. It is an autoimmune condition in which the body's immune system mistakenly identifies proteins within the thyroid as foreign. The thyroid gland is slowly destroyed over time.

- Symptoms of Hashimoto's thyroiditis often occur after the autoimmune process has been active for at least a year, often longer. The onset of classic hypothyroid symptoms indicate significant damage to the thyroid gland has occurred.

- The development of Hashimoto's thyroiditis occurs among those who are genetically susceptible but only in the presence of a triggering event. Triggers may include viruses, intestinal infections, hormonal changes, environmental toxins, and radiation exposure.

- During the course of Hashimoto's thyroiditis symptoms can include hyperthyroid symptoms along with hypothyroid symptoms as the thyroid tissue destruction releases pockets of stored thyroid hormones.

- Supplementing with iodine is controversial in functional medicine. Some practitioners believe use will worsening autoimmune thyroid conditions, while others use high dose iodine as a therapy in Hashimoto's thyroiditis.

- Low-dose naltrexone is a revolutionary new therapy that can reduce the antibodies of autoimmune diseases. The use of LDN may be of value for anyone with Hashimoto's thyroiditis.

CHAPTER 5

Liver, Digestion, and Adrenals

THIS CHAPTER FOCUSES ON THE INTERPLAY between the thyroid and different organ systems. Organs such as the liver, digestive tract, and adrenal glands influence thyroid function and are influenced in turn. For example, the liver is one of the main sites for thyroid hormone conversion; if the liver is functioning poorly, conversion will suffer.

Similarly, low thyroid function strongly influences the digestive system, resulting in poor nutrient absorption and an increased chance of intestinal infections due to parasites, viruses, or harmful bacteria. The digestive tract can also be a trigger for autoimmune thyroid conditions caused by an overgrowth of certain species of bacteria.

The adrenals are especially important because they, along with the thyroid, play a critical role in the complex interplay of the endocrine system. Often, low thyroid function and either under- or overactive adrenal function are seen together. This combination often occurs when individuals undergo significant periods of stress. The adrenals become overactive which suppresses thyroid function.

When there is dysfunction in one or more of these organ systems, which is common, it needs to be addressed or else it may disrupt proper thyroid function. Addressing such dysfunction ranges across treating leaky gut, clearing out autoimmune-causing intestinal infections (in the case of Hashimoto's), and correcting high cortisol output from the adrenal glands to lower high rT3.

The important thing to remember is that there are ways of testing each of these areas to directly pinpoint what's going on and develop a proper treatment plan. In some cases, simple blood tests can give us the insight we need, other times more advanced functional medicine tests are needed to uncover the cause of dysfunction. In this chapter, we'll review all of these issues, the best tests to use, and the key points to correct the problem.

Liver Dysfunction and Thyroid Conversion Problems

The liver has long been a focus of naturopathic medicine. Naturopathic physicians recognize that reduced liver function can either cause or contribute to numerous health problems. The liver has many roles in the body, including that of the chief recycler and detoxifier.

Every substance that enters the bloodstream passes through and, to some degree, is processed by the liver through the phase one and two detoxification pathways. In phase one, liver enzymes reduce the toxicity of substances through a process called oxidation-reduction and hydrolysis. This first step removes some of the toxicity of the substance being processed. In phase two, these toxins are further processed.

In ideal circumstances the liver correctly processes everything it encounters; toxins are neutralized, old proteins and cholesterol are recycled, and nutrients are further broken down and either stored or packaged for other tissues. Unfortunately, in today's toxic world we no longer live in ideal circumstances.

While liver disease such as hepatitis and fatty liver will result in structural damage to the liver and the associated decreased liver function, such damage is not the only cause of reduced liver function. It should also be noted that the cause-and-effect relationship is mutual: decreased functionality of the liver often leads to structural changes - but that is outside the scope of this book.

We now turn to what is often referred to as liver congestion, an overworked liver, often overwhelmed by the toxins it is exposed to daily from a variety of sources including pollution, medications, poor diet, intestinal infections, and compounded by a lack of exercise. This results in a decrease in liver function.

Remembering that every cell in the body depends on thyroid hormone to function. If low thyroid function occurs, either from hypothyroidism or another cause, we will see liver function decrease even further. This decidedly vicious cycle can diminish the capacity of the liver to convert T4 into T3.

Not only can pollution decrease overall liver function, environmental toxins such as Bisphenol-A (BPA), used in plastic water bottles and as a liner of canned foods, can block T4 to T3 conversion by radically reducing the function of the deiodinase D1 enzyme, which is found in high concentrations in the liver.

Toxins with similar effects include mercury, pesticides, and Polybrominated Diphenyl Ether (PBDE), a flame-retardant used in clothing, mattresses, carpeting, and car interiors. The levels of these toxins are highest in the United States, and especially in California as indicated by research showing a fourfold increase compared to other states.

In addition to toxins compromising liver function, there are classes of toxic substances that directly affect thyroid hormone conversion, such as flame retardants, rocket fuel, and pesticides. All of these factors can contribute to liver congestion and sluggish detox pathways.

Again, when we confront low thyroid function we must consider the current health of the liver and its toxic exposure. In most, there will be some degree of dysfunction. My intention is not to paint a picture of "doom and gloom." I assure you, there is much you can do to improve liver detox pathways. Even by simply limiting your pesticide exposure in your diet, as discussed later in Chapter 9, you can improve your overall health, specifically the thyroid hormone conversion process.

So, how do you know if you have liver congestion? There are clues to indicate reduced liver function. Symptoms include acne or eczema, moodiness, poor sleep, chemical sensitivities, hormone imbalances, and gallbladder problems.

- Skin problems such as acne or eczema may be the result of the body trying to eliminate through the skin toxins that the liver was unable to clear from the bloodstream. As the liver recycles old hormones, a buildup of such hormones may be another cause of acne or eczema.

- Moodiness – irritability, anger, and depression – has long been associated with diminished liver function in Chinese medicine. A 2017 study from China was one among several studies in recent years that have found evidence that demonstrates a relationship between liver disease and depression.

- Poor sleep – either trouble falling asleep or staying asleep – is often an effect of liver congestion. Metabolites, normally eliminated, build up, enter circulation, trigger inflammation in the brain, and disrupt the sleep/wake cycle.

- Chemical sensitivities have long been associated with overwhelmed liver detox pathways. Normally, the body would process these chemicals with little or no symptoms presented. The inability of the congested liver to process these chemicals results in symptoms, such as headaches, anxiety, and dizziness.

- The liver plays two important roles in hormone regulation. First, it creates and secretes important hormones such as Insulin-like Growth Factor-1 (IGF) and Angiotensinogen (which helps regulate blood pressure). Liver congestion can hinder proper hormone production and secretion, which, in turn, weakens/undermines the endocrine system. Second, the liver recycles sex hormones such as estrogen, progesterone, and testosterone. In this case, the congested liver is unable to break down these hormones resulting in a buildup in the body.

- Gallbladder disorders often begin in the liver, which creates the bile that is stored in the gallbladder. When the liver is not functioning properly, it can change the amount, and/or the consistency of the bile produced. It becomes thicker, and gallbladder stones are more likely to form. Fatty food intolerance and right upper abdominal pain are hallmarks of gallbladder dysfunction.

Overall liver and gallbladder health can be assessed through basic blood tests, such as liver enzymes and other blood markers. However, special tests are needed to determine how effective the liver detoxification pathways are working. There are several approaches to testing, all of which are effective. Among my favorite is the Organic Acids panel by Genova Diagnostics. I discuss this in more detail in chapter 7.

Disease Begins in the Digestive Tract

The importance of a healthy digestive tract was recognized long ago. Hippocrates, the ancient Greek physician, was quoted as saying, "All disease begins in the gut." What was true 2500 years ago remains true today. In fact, research has now uncovered just how right Hippocrates was.

Why Look at Your Digestive Function?

It is remarkable to consider the negative impact that poor digestion has on the absorption of nutrients and the deficiencies and anemias that can result. Adding to the concern is the fact that infections and inflammation in the gut are becoming more common.

When we look at any system of the body, we commonly find external influences. The digestive tract is no different. We will look at several examples of gastrointestinal disorders to see how they ultimately influence the thyroid.

How Well Does Your Digestion Work?

It is common to experience sluggish digestion with thyroid conditions that reduce the amount of active thyroid hormone in the digestive system. It can be a challenge to determine which came first, the digestive disorder or the thyroid disorder. While constipation is the most common symptom of low thyroid function, other gastrointestinal symptoms can occur, including diarrhea, bloating, and gas, all of which may be due to poor absorption or opportunistic infections.

If you have any digestive symptoms, it is wise to examine further to determine the cause. This section will review the most common causes, contributing factors, and results of low thyroid function.

Parasympathetic Nervous System: Rest and Digest

Before starting off on an "A to Z" tour of the digestive tract and how it works, it is best to begin before we start eating. Our mental and emotional state when we eat is important. Our body needs to be relaxed when eating. There are two parts of the nervous system we will focus on in this section. The sympathetic part, commonly called the fight-or-flight part of the nervous system, helped early humans survive the threat of predators and other dangers. The parasympathetic portion, referred to as the rest-

and-digest part, should be dominant when we eat and sleep. With our modern, fast-paced, high-stress lifestyle the sympathetic fight-or-flight wins out.

Just look at the popularity of fast food, the prevalence of the 30-minute lunch, and all the people hurrily eating breakfast on their way to work. These are not healthy parasympathetic situations.

Because so many of us eat our meals in varying degrees of stress, we eat our food faster and more of it because we don't give our body enough time to register fullness. As a result, our digestive tracts are not able to break down the food we eat.

Furthermore, I rarely see people chew their food adequately. Many natural health experts recommend chewing each bite 32 times. The number 32 is arbitrary but should enough to nearly liquify the food so that the enzymes in the saliva can break down the food even more. This will allow the stomach to process the food faster.

Based on my observations, most people chew each bite about three to five times. That's far from sufficient. One indication that you aren't chewing your food enough is a need to drink fluids with your meals. This is common, and I often see people drinking cold drinks, which is even worse!

Stomach, Stomach Acid, and Breaking Down Food

After chewing your food (I recommend, at least, ten times) the food travels down the esophagus into the stomach. The stomach consists of 3 layers of muscles that squeeze and mash the food to help break it down further. The stomach also produces acid that helps break down proteins and other food types. The pH is very acidic, around 2.0. This acid also helps protect the body from harmful bacteria, much like a moat around a castle.

I find that some patients have a low amount of stomach acid, often due to chronic stress driving the sympathetic nervous system into overdrive. When the sympathetic nervous system is overactive, the blood and nerve flow is directed away from the digestive tract, which reduces the amount of stomach acid produced. In this case, the food, not broken down properly, tends to sit in the stomach longer than it should. Furthermore, when stomach acid production is reduced, the small intestine is not prepared to receive the food in the next step.

Small Intestine - The Important Role of Nutrient Absorption

Once food has been broken down by the stomach, it enters the small intestine, which immediately neutralizes the acid by releasing sodium bicarbonate, as alkaline as stomach acid is acidic. When the small intestine reacts to the presence of food it also triggers the release of bile from the gallbladder to help break down fats.

Simultaneously, the pancreas releases pancreatic enzymes to help break down the food into small particles that the small intestine cells can absorb. The primary role of the small intestine is to absorb nutrients. Its secondary function is to fight off sources of potential infection in what we consume. In fact, the small and large intestine constitute 70% of the immune system.

Intestinal permeability, also known as leaky gut syndrome, can occur when the surface cells of the small intestine become damaged. Many substances cause this damage, including antibiotics, NSAIDs (aspirin, ibuprofen, etc.), antacids, harmful bacteria, yeast, viruses, food additives, and foods such as gluten.

With leaky gut, gaps form in the otherwise tight interlinking cell surface of the small intestine, allowing particles of food, microbes, and other substances to enter deep into the intestinal tissue. There the immune system encounters these particles and marks them as foreign invaders. This can trigger food reactivities and allergies. The immune system may also go into overdrive, recruiting more immune cells into the area, which can decrease the small intestine's ability to absorb nutrients.

Whenever I encounter a patient who is likely to have intestinal permeability, I rely on the Advance Intestinal Barrier Assessment panel by Dunwoody Labs, which I find to be invaluable. The test looks for markers found in intestinal permeability, such as zonulin, histamine, and lipopolysaccharides, which indicate that bacteria has penetrated deep into the tissues and that inflammation is increasing in the small intestine. Such inflammation increases the risk of autoimmune disease conditions, including Hashimoto's thyroiditis.

Once the cause of intestinal permeability is discovered, a treatment plan can be devised to seal up the spaces between the cells, heal the intestinal tissue, reduce inflammation, and the reactivity of the immune system. If intestinal permeability is present, this is a crucial step to take. Thankfully, functional medicine practitioners have these helpful tools at their disposal to detect and correct intestinal permeability.

Intestinal Microbial Imbalance

The relationship between the thyroid and the digestive tract is a complicated one. As with all tissues in the body, the cells of the gastrointestinal tract are dependent on thyroid hormone to regulate the level of cellular activity, aka metabolism. With low levels of thyroid hormone, one commonly associates a slow digestive tract with poor absorption and constipation, both classic symptoms of hypothyroidism. But a closer look will reveal greater complexity.

When the intestinal microbiome is out of balance, with fewer healthy bacteria and higher amounts of unhealthy microbes, the condition is called dysbiosis. When dysbiosis occurs in the gut, the thyroid conversion process in the intestines will be significantly reduced. Some species of bacteria release a toxin that triggers inflammation in the intestines and can spread to other parts of the body.

Inflammation, as I've mentioned before, can reduce the effectiveness of thyroid hormone conversion, and cause the thyroid feedback loop in the brain (hypothalamus and pituitary) to become less active. Furthermore, other bacterial species within the dysbiotic spectrum are known to trigger autoimmunity, in some cases, Hashimoto's thyroiditis.

My approach to treating the thyroid condition is to look at the overall health picture. As you may know, the digestive tract – which includes the liver – is essential. In searching for the cause of low thyroid function, including autoimmune thyroid conditions such as Hashimoto's thyroiditis, it is essential to recognize the vital role that digestive imbalance plays, both as a cause and a contributing factor, in worsening thyroid conditions.

The Role of Intestinal Bacteria in Thyroid Problems

Research into the bacteria found in the large intestine referred to collectively as the microbiome, has been ongoing for years. The latest information indicates that these bacteria help determine our health because they have a massive impact on nutrient absorption and regulation of hormones.

Also, they influence approximately 20% of thyroid hormone conversion. The gut microbes help convert T4 into T3 sulfate, a molecule similar to T3. A unique enzyme called intestinal sulfatase, found in healthy intestinal tracts and produced by healthy gut bacteria, helps convert T3 sulfatase into the more metabolically active T3.

Bile, created by the liver, released by the gallbladder, and helpful in breaking down fat, influences thyroid hormone conversion as well. After bile breaks down dietary fats in the small intestine, it travels to the large intestine and is converted by bacteria into what is called secondary bile acids.

Depending on your gut health, these can form into healthy bile acids when converted by healthy gut bacteria or into unhealthy bile acids when bad gut bacteria and yeast have overrun the good bacteria. This distinction is important because healthy secondary bile acids are needed to help with the thyroid conversion process.

Do You Have Parasites or an Intestinal Infection?

Did you know that gut infections can be a trigger for autoimmune thyroid disease? As it turns out, there are certain bacteria that can be a trigger for many autoimmune conditions, including Hashimoto's thyroiditis and the hyperthyroid condition, Graves' disease. There are a number of autoimmune-triggering infections found in the digestive tract.

The process of a virus or bacteria triggering an autoimmune disease occurs through molecular mimicry. According to the theory, the immune system becomes confused and attacks thyroid cells, mistaking the proteins on the surface of these cells for the protein on bacteria and other microbial invaders. Ultimately, it's a case of mistaken identity. To illustrate the process, I will provide a few examples of bacteria known to cause molecular mimicry:

- Helicobacter pylori (H. pylori) is bacteria found in the stomach that causes stomach ulcers and occasionally stomach cancer. It also depletes stomach acid, which hinders digestion. Low stomach acid may also influence the absorption of your supplements and medications. The exact mechanism isn't clear, but studies have repeatedly found those with autoimmune thyroiditis were twice as likely to have an H. pylori infection than those without thyroid antibodies. More importantly, further research found a reduction in TPO antibodies after successfully eradicating H. pylori infections.

- Pseudomonas aeruginosa is commonly found in the large intestine and is well behaved in a colon with a healthy balance of intestinal flora, but it can become quite nasty when the body experiences high stress or trauma. In fact, it can turn deadly if it bores through the intestinal wall and into the bloodstream. Additionally, Pseudomonas aeruginosa has been found to trigger celiac disease in those who are genetically susceptible as it contains a high number of enzymes that quickly break down gluten from wheat. These bacteria can also carry gluten particles deep into the tissues of the small intestine and thus potentially trigger thyroid autoimmunity molecular mimicry through immune reactivity to gluten.

- Klebsiella pneumoniae is another potent autoimmune trigger that has been linked to ankylosing spondylitis, inflammatory bowel disease, and Hashimoto's thyroiditis in genetically susceptible individuals. It does not typically present significant digestive symptoms. In fact, the most common symptoms reported with klebsiella overgrowth are brain fog, fatigue, and joint pain.

- Yersinia enterocolitica has one of the strongest associations with autoimmune thyroid because TSH binds to the surface of this bacteria! This significantly increases the risk of an immune attack on thyroid peroxidase enzymes and thyroglobulin because the immune system will associate thyroid proteins with this bacteria in another case of mistaken identity.

The Best Tests for Parasites and Infections

Comprehensive stool testing has existed for several decades and can be useful in determining your overall digestive health. Since I've been in practice, however, there has been a shift. The process now includes testing for genetic markers of microbes found in the gut.

In my opinion, the most useful test is the GI-MAP stool test by Diagnostic Laboratories. Using the latest DNA technology, this test looks for DNA strands from bacteria, yeasts, parasites, worms, and viruses. This makes results even more accurate because the lab no longer needs to grow a microbe culture or find parasite eggs. Another benefit of this technology is that it can determine the severity of an infection.

Small Intestinal Bacterial Overgrowth

Remember how I mentioned that low thyroid hormone levels hamper gut function? Diminished digestive function entails reduced absorption of essential nutrients and extended transit time in the intestines, meaning that food will begin to ferment in the intestines. That's bad news.

In the small intestine, this snowball effect can lead to bacteria colonizing an otherwise microbe-free environment. These bacteria – which are often healthy bacteria in the large intestine – feed on the undigested food in the small intestine and thrive there.

Normally, the small intestine has mechanisms that prevent bacterial colonization, but in this case, I've been describing the nerves of the intestines aren't as active due to the reduced amount of thyroid hormone reaching the intestines. This condition, commonly referred to as Small Intestinal Bacterial Overgrowth (SIBO), is both caused by and an exacerbating factor of low thyroid function.

Whenever a patient with thyroid symptoms also experiences symptoms of nausea, reflux, gas, abdominal bloating, and constipation, I suspect SIBO. These symptoms are associated with the hydrogen or methane gas that is the waste product of these bacteria colonies. Not everyone with digestive symptoms has SIBO, but it is often worth further investigation.

Typically, I order a SIBO breath test which indicates if there is an overgrowth of bacteria in the small intestine. Positive results also show where in the small bowel this is occurring. The breath test does not indicate which species of bacteria are in the small intestine, however. Conversely, a comprehensive stool test will tell you what microbes are found in the intestines, but not where they are located. Using both tests when appropriate can give you a clear picture of intestinal health.

Adrenal Fatigue Syndrome and Low Thyroid

The adrenal glands, which sit atop the kidneys, are part of the endocrine system. The adrenals produce several types of hormones. We are going to focus on cortisol, commonly called the stress hormone, though its role encompasses more than just stress. The hormone production activity of the adrenal glands is controlled by the hypothalamus and pituitary gland, two other primary components of the endocrine system. The interaction between these three glands is referred to as the Hypothalamic-Pituitary-Adrenal Axis (HPA). Much like the relationship of the Hypothalamic-Pituitary-Thyroid axis (HPT), the adrenal output is subject to changes in parts of the endocrine system. As an example, low thyroid activity may result in increased adrenal hormone production as means of compensation. Understanding the role of cortisol in the body is essential because high or low cortisol levels can negatively impact several critical areas in the thyroid process.

Cortisol levels fluctuate throughout the day. Following a 24-hour circadian rhythm, they are highest in the morning and lowest at night. Cortisol is a glucocorticoid steroid, which means that it helps regulate blood sugar levels by triggering the production of glucose (blood sugar) from proteins inside the liver. It also helps cells use fat as energy within the cells.

Additionally, cortisol has an crucial anti-inflammatory role in the body and helps reduce the damage that inflammation can cause in the body. The adrenal glands will produce higher amounts of cortisol during periods of high stress and inflammation. During emergencies, the adrenal glands will release a burst of cortisol along with adrenaline as a part of the "fight or flight" portion of the nervous system. There are undesirable consequences of elevated cortisol levels; the most noticeable effect is weight gain.

Certain adrenal gland diseases can destroy the ability to produce cortisol (Addison's disease). Particular tumor growths can cause an overproduction of cortisol (Cushing's disease). We're not going to focus on those conditions. Instead, we're going to set our sights between these two extremes and look at adrenal dysfunction, commonly called Adrenal Fatigue syndrome.

Adrenal Fatigue syndrome is a condition in which chronic stress and inflammation alter cortisol production. There are four distinct stages of Adrenal Fatigue Syndrome.

Adrenal Fatigue Syndrome and Chronic Stress

Stage 1: Alarm Reaction

In the first stage, called the alarm reaction, cortisol is higher than normal due to high stress. In the beginning of stage one people usually feel pretty good, but often need some type of stimulant, such as caffeine, to get them started in the morning. I believe caffeine's pride of place in modern culture illustrates, at least in part, how common stage one adrenal fatigue really is.

Most people will be in stage one for short periods of major stress, such as moving, starting a new job, or an emergency. After the source of stress diminishes, healthy individuals will recover with rest.

Stage 2 - Resistance

Those who experience ongoing stressors often also experience exacerbated Adrenal Fatigue Syndrome (AFS) symptoms. In most cases, symptoms of stage 2 are mild with increased fatigue, which most people address with a second or third cup of coffee.

Elevated cortisol increases appetite and brings on sugar cravings. Overeating, especially high carbohydrate foods, results in abdominal obesity, often described as an "apple shape" body type. In stage 2, it is common to see higher cholesterol and borderline high blood pressure because the adrenals will also produce adrenaline (aka epinephrine), which will constrict the arteries as a response to stress.

Because cortisol release is meant to follow a 24-hour circadian rhythm, continuously elevated cortisol production requires more resources than the adrenal glands can spare. The body will steal resources from other systems to ensure cortisol production can be maintained.

After an extended period of increased cortisol production, the adrenal glands resort to using the hormone precursor, pregnenolone, to continue to make more cortisol. Normally, pregnenolone produces several sex hormones, including progesterone and dehydroepiandrosterone (DHEA).

DHEA is a sex hormone precursor, capable of making both estrogen and testosterone. The body will gladly sacrifice the sex hormones to ensure cortisol levels are high enough to deal with the inflammation. Because the adrenals are using pregnenolone for cortisol production, progesterone and DHEA levels begin to decline.

Commonly women will experience symptoms of low progesterone, such as increased PMS, fluid retention, and weight gain, especially around the abdomen, buttocks, and thighs. A person can stay in stage two for months or even years so long as the adrenal glands can produce enough cortisol.

The elevated cortisol associated with stage 2 will begin to affect thyroid function. Commonly we will see the onset of thyroid hormone conversion problems with an increase in reverse T3 production and reduced conversion to T3. Both the increased inflammation and the cortisol produced to address the inflammation can upset the balance of the hypothalamus, altering its sensitivity to the amount of circulating thyroid hormone. Finally, elevated cortisol can precipitate thyroid hormone resistance at a cellular level.

Many people will spend most of their lives in stage 2 without moving into stage 3. People in stage 2 can recover with extra rest, exercise, better stress management, and changes in dietary habits, like cutting out sugar.

Stage 3 - Adrenal Exhaustion

Those who progress to stage 3 often experience massive ongoing stressors. Some of the most common situations that provoke stage 3 Adrenal Fatigue include working in the medical field (especially working long or overnight shifts), high-stress jobs, such as emergency responder, and juggling the responsibilities of parenthood, especially with three or more children.

For most people stage 3 begins when the adrenal glands fail to keep up with the demand for cortisol due to the depletion of key nutrients such as vitamin B5, vitamin C, zinc, and magnesium. As a result, cortisol levels decline. Subsequently, without enough cortisol to keep it under control, the chronic stress-associated inflammation spikes.

Progesterone and DHEA levels continue to drop, and we see more noticeable hormonal symptoms, ranging from severe premenstrual tension (PMS) to low fertility. Signs of fatigue worsen considerably, ranging from end-of-the-day exhaustion to complete immobilization. Insomnia, often described as "wired and tired," is another common symptom of stage 3.

Weight begins to shift from uncontrolled gain to loss. Many in stage 3 struggle to keep weight on, especially muscle mass. Chronic muscle weakness and reduced endurance are common.

The thyroid is also strongly affected in stage 3 because low cortisol will reduce thyroid hormone conversion and cause decreased thyroid hormone cellular receptor activity, resulting in less T3 hormone entering into and activating the metabolism of the cells.

Stage 4 - Adrenal Failure

In stage 4, the adrenals and the regulatory efforts of the hypothalamus and pituitary are incapable of dealing with any stress. The system has virtually shut down. The symptoms of stage 4 are so severe that they are practically indistinguishable from Addison's disease. People in this state are bedridden and often hospitalized. Addressing all the complications of this late-stage condition is well out of the scope of this book. An endocrinologist typically manages adrenal failure.

Testing for Adrenal Fatigue Syndrome

Conventional medical practitioners typically order blood tests when looking for signs of severe adrenal diseases, such as Addison's or Cushing's diseases. Unfortunately, when testing for adrenal fatigue syndrome, these blood tests are not sensitive enough to detect the changes we want to track.

However, testing saliva for cortisol and DHEA levels is both effective and inexpensive. In the functional medicine community, the Adrenal Stress Index test, a 12-hour saliva collection that measures cortisol and DHEA, is considered the "gold standard" for measuring Adrenal Fatigue syndrome. Over the 12 hours, most tests will collect four samples of saliva, morning, noon, afternoon, and evening.

Having four distinct collection times helps determine the health of the cortisol circadian rhythm. There is an established daily range for cortisol levels: morning is the highest, with a gradual decline through the afternoon and into night time, which sees the lowest cortisol levels. DHEA, measured in two of the four samples, is averaged to determine if its levels are where they should be.

Other forms of testing are becoming popular, including urine adrenal tests, which are especially useful because they measure both the adrenals and the sex hormones. I often use the D.U.T.C.H. test by Precision Analytics which uses dried urine samples to detect adrenal and sex hormone imbalances.

Chapter Highlights

- The liver is a major site of thyroid hormone conversion which is negatively impacted when the liver detoxification pathways are functioning poorly or are overwhelmed with toxins. Environmental toxins, poor diet, and inflammation can reduce liver function.

- Digestive disorders can both cause of and are caused by low thyroid function. Nutrient malabsorption is common and results in worsening of symptoms.

- Intestinal bacteria help convert T4 to the active T3 hormone. Intestinal microbe imbalances or infections can impede this process.

- Certain species of pathogenic bacteria can trigger many autoimmune conditions, including Hashimoto's thyroiditis. There are advanced stool tests that detect these bacteria and any other type of digestive tract infection.

- Adrenal Fatigue Syndrome (AFS) is commonly triggered by prolonged stress or inflammation. Low thyroid function is often worsened by the altered cortisol production associated with AFS.

CHAPTER 6

Why Thyroid Disorders Are Not Treated Effectively

The Narrow Perspective of Conventional Medicine

AS I HAVE MENTIONED EARLIER IN THIS BOOK, modern healthcare has made incredible advances in fields of medicine that provide lifesaving treatments and therapies. Unfortunately, it has not made comparable strides in the field of thyroid medicine and treatment. Conventional medicine only recognizes one illness associated with low thyroid hormone, hypothyroidism, and its only approach to hypothyroidism is providing thyroid hormone replacement in the form of levothyroxine, which is the synthetic form of T4.

Conventional medicine practitioners look for one thing: evidence that the thyroid is not producing enough thyroid hormone. Their answer is to provide T4 medication to fill the gap between what the thyroid can produce and what the body needs. Most practitioners do not focus on the cause of poor thyroid function, and even if they do, they rarely have anything to offer other than T4 medication.

The use of T4-only medication has its issues as discussed below. As you've seen by now, low thyroid hormone may spawn a whole host of conditions, each calling for its own particular treatment plan. As we will see below, many patients do not experience as much benefit from T4-only medication as one would hope. Also, since most practitioners use limited testing – the typical TSH-only test protocol – they not only fail to recognize the other forms of low-thyroid hormone disorders but also may prescribe the T4 medication at too low of a dosage.

Furthermore, conventional medicine's limited approach to reduced thyroid function does not account for possible nutritional deficiencies, which may be having a detrimental effect. Allowing such deficiencies to continue untreated may compromise the efficiency of the medication as the nutrients needed to convert T4 and to make energy in the cell may be missing. Medication alone is simply not enough to address all possible factors regarding thyroid related disorders.

Outdated Mechanical Thinking

The current body of knowledge about thyroid disorders is quite vast, but the current medical model of thyroid dysfunction as seen in the typical clinical setting is based on an outdated, mechanical concept of the thyroid as simply being broken, which fails to recognize the interconnectedness of the endocrine system. Moreover, it fails to acknowledge the harmful effects of chronic illness, nutritional deficiencies, and inflammation of the thyroid gland, the sites of thyroid hormone conversion, and cellular activity of thyroid hormones.

Is the Thyroid Really "Broken"?

This is a fundamental question, and in most cases, my answer is no. To be clear, the term "broken" as it relates to thyroid would imply that the thyroid is no longer capable of producing adequate thyroid hormone without outside intervention. Conventional medical thinking is that the thyroid is indeed broken when a patient is diagnosed as being hypothyroid and the conclusion is that thyroid hormone replacement is the best bet for a long-term solution. I think their best bet is a bad bet, and here's why:

1. The thyroid gland tissue is capable of regenerating new cells to replace damaged cells. There are limits to this growth, but it is possible. There are instances, such as surgical removal and long-term autoimmune thyroid damage, in which the thyroid has too much scar tissue to repair itself.

2. The autoimmune process of thyroiditis can be slowed, stopped, and potentially reversed. The destruction of tissue caused by white blood cells attacking the thyroid is the primary cause of hypothyroidism in the modern industrialized world, and it is considered a "one-way ticket" to thyroid failure by conventional medicine. However, provided that the conditions that trigger the autoimmune response are removed, the autoimmune process will typically stop, and the regenerative process of the thyroid can begin. Hashimoto's thyroiditis triggered by intestinal infection is a good example.

3. Thyroid efficiency is subject to outside influences. The ability to produce thyroid hormone can be affected by the level of inflammation in the body, cortisol interference, and vitamin and mineral deficiencies.

The Limitations of Relying on TSH Lab Testing Only

I first suspected something just wasn't right regarding TSH testing early on in my career when I found that patients continued to experience symptoms of low thyroid function when I would prescribe and adjust medication to normalize the elevated TSH lab result. As I came to understand the thyroid better, I expanded my lab testing to a functional perspective.

Later in my career, I had a patient who went to have the thyroid blood tests I had ordered (including TSH, of course) drawn one morning around 9 am. She just happened to be participating in a thyroid study at a local medical university that required her to get periodically drawn for TSH, which she did an hour later. When I saw the two results side by side, I was blown away. Within 60 minutes her TSH had decreased 40% of the lab range!

If the TSH test was truly the foundational piece of the thyroid medicine, as it had always been regarded, such a significant change should not have happened, especially within an hour. So, what happened in this hour between the two draws? She had eaten. The first draw was on an empty stomach, and she was even feeling a bit woozy afterward. As it turns out, research has found that food consumption can influence your TSH level.

What's more, it is well established that the pituitary production and excretion of TSH changes throughout the day as the process has its own circadian (24-hour) rhythm. Can you guess when TSH is the most active? At night! Studies find that the thyroid is more active at night due to the pituitary stimulation through increased TSH. This makes sense: during the night the body more frequently shifts into repair and replace mode. TSH levels are highest in the morning and slowly decreases throughout the day. This means morning draws are more accurate.

The Problems with T4-Only Therapy

The medication levothyroxine is the synthetic form of thyroxine (T4) and is the medication of choice for the treatment of hypothyroidism in the conventional medical world. As of 2015, levothyroxine was the most commonly prescribed medication in the U.S., with 21 million prescriptions that year. This would suggest that a significant number of people seem to experience relief of their hypothyroid symptoms with this medication.

This does not account for everyone, however, since approximately 25%-30% of those treated with levothyroxine continue to experience ongoing symptoms of hypothyroidism. Based on my experience this percentage is more likely about 40%. There is a growing patient-driven movement, including the "Stop the Thyroid Madness" group, which is focused on addressing the limitations of T4-only therapy.

T4 Conversion Issues

For many, reality differs quite dramatically from what they hear about their thyroid in a typical clinical setting. Several studies have found that many of the patients on a T4-only therapy had lower T3 hormone in their blood than did the control group consisting of healthy individuals who didn't have thyroid conditions. If T4 medication worked as promised, you would expect that the medication would be converting from T4 to T3 correctly and that T3 blood levels would match those of the healthy test subjects. The research shows that many of the thyroid subjects were converting poorly, which would explain the ongoing low thyroid symptoms.

Another justification for using T4-only is that it is "safer" than using T3. Much of this reasoning comes from research from the 1950s, which suffered from inaccurate testing. New research finds that T3 medication can play a useful role in treatment. It is interesting to note that there are no side effects listed for T3 medication. The only symptoms that one can experience relate to excessive intake, which is simple to remedy.

TSH Is Used to Monitor T4 Replacement

Ongoing symptoms may be related to misleading TSH levels. Due to TSH levels fluctuating, as described above, prescribed dosage may be too low. Furthermore, individuals in such cases are often those who are more likely to experience thyroid hormone conversion problems based on genetics, nutrient deficiencies, inflammation, or a combination of two or more of these factors.

T4 Medication May Trigger Weight Gain

In my years of working with thyroid patients, I have noticed that some patients seem to gain weight when taking levothyroxine (T4-only) therapy. My first thought was that they undermedicated or that thyroid hormone conversion was compromised. But as I investigated this further, I came across a book by Kenneth Blanchard MD, titled *Functional Approach to Hypothyroidism: Bridging Traditional and Alternative Treatment Approaches for Total Patient Wellness*. In the book, Dr. Blanchard reveals that taking levothyroxine on an empty stomach increases hunger.

It is his theory that when the T4 medication comes in contact with stomach lining, it triggers the release of the hormones that regulate hunger and weight gain. Dr. Blanchard recommends taking T4 medication with food. Keep in mind that doing so can interfere with the absorption of the medication, but this is easily remedied by increasing the dosage to compensate for the lost effectiveness.

T4 May Work Better at Night

As mentioned above, TSH begins to rise about 2 hours before we go to bed. As TSH rises, the thyroid starts releasing T4 to facilitate repairs in the body as we sleep. It is for this reason that some practitioners recommend taking thyroid medication at night. This is especially pertinent if sleep is restless. Many who make the switch find that they sleep better when they take their T4 medication with dinner.

Please note that this applies specifically to T4-only medication. Many find that the T3 can be too stimulating, compromising sleep quality. As such, it is suggested that T3 and desiccated (T4/T3 combo) medications be taken in the morning or in the late afternoon.

Why Thyroid Conditions are So Commonly Missed

Because of the massive impact that low thyroid hormone can have on the body, symptoms vary widely from person to person. Fatigue is the most common of the thyroid symptoms, but symptoms also include anxiousness, insomnia, muscle aches, joint pain, water retention, abdominal bloating, headaches, and poor memory, to name a few.

Low thyroid function is often misdiagnosed as a mood disorder, such as depression, anxiety disorder, or mood swings. Women with low thyroid function who are diagnosed with a mood disorder are more likely experiencing premenstrual syndrome (PMS), which is usually treated with birth control.

Fibromyalgia or other muscle or joint disorders are common in thyroid conditions, especially in thyroid hormone conversion disorders.

Another common condition seen with low thyroid function is Raynaud's syndrome in which arteries in the hand constrict, cutting off blood supply. Raynaud's is triggered by cold exposure and has been described as an "allergy to the cold." Not everyone with Raynaud's syndrome has thyroid problems but the overlap between these two conditions is significant.

Another excellent example of misdiagnosis is irritable bowel syndrome (IBS), a condition in which gas, bloating, cramps, constipation, and/or diarrhea is experienced after eating. I have worked with patients who could only overcome their IBS once their thyroid function was corrected.

Looking closer at depression, I commonly see patients who have obvious low thyroid conditions but were diagnosed as being depressed. The diagnostic guidelines for depression explicitly state that other possible causes, such as hypothyroidism, should be tested and ruled out before giving an antidepressant. Many practitioners treat in the reverse order: doing an antidepressant trial first and a testing second (if at all).

Depression medication has its place, and no doubt has been life-saving for those who are genuinely depressed. That said, it is essential to rule out any form of thyroid disorder before making the diagnosis of depression, as proper diagnosis is fundamental to the practice of medicine.

Chapter Highlights

- Conventional medicine practitioners look for one thing: evidence that the thyroid is not producing enough thyroid hormone. Their answer is to provide T4 medication.

- The current clinical model is an outdated, mechanical concept of the thyroid as simply being broken, which fails to recognize the interconnectedness of the endocrine system.

- TSH-only testing fails to take into account the impacts of nutrient deficiency and inflammation within the thyroid system. This testing method is based on the mechanistic thinking of conventional medicine.

- T4-only replacement therapy fails to address thyroid hormone conversion issues and often results in partial improvement of low thyroid symptoms.

- Low thyroid symptoms can be varied due to the number of body systems that can be negatively impacted. Low thyroid function is often misdiagnosed as a mood disorder, such as depression, anxiety disorder, or mood swings.

CHAPTER 7

How to Get Tested Correctly

Using Lab Tests to Determine Thyroid Function

AS I HAVE STATED PREVIOUSLY IT IS IMPORTANT to test more than TSH when evaluating the thyroid. In this chapter, we will look at the thyroid labs tests I recommend and why these tests provide a clearer picture. In addition, I will discuss some of the patterns you might see in lab results, and some do's and don'ts of testing, including how to proceed if you encounter resistance from your healthcare provider.

Preparation For Testing

Getting a blood test is simple. Getting accurate results can be more of a challenge. There are a multitude of factors that can falsely raise or lower thyroid lab results. Here are some guidelines for maximizing the accuracy of your lab results.

72 hours: Stop All Biotin

Biotin, vitamin B7, has become a popular supplement to help trigger hair growth. It works well, and I recommend it frequently to my patients.

The downside is that the same dose that may restore a full head of hair can wreak havoc on your thyroid lab results. This happens because of the way that labs measure thyroid hormone blood samples. Part of the process uses biotin in measuring TSH, thyroid hormones, and thyroid antibody levels. The amount of biotin you get from food isn't nearly enough to influence these tests, but the higher doses found in these hair growth supplements are enough to radically alter your results.

For example, biotin supplementation is likely to falsely elevate free T4 and free T3 levels and lower TSH, giving the impression that you have hyperthyroidism (Graves' disease) or that your dosage is way too high! Even worse it can elevate TSH receptor antibodies, which is another indicator of Graves' disease! Based on these false premises, your doctor may lower your medication or misdiagnose you.

The simple solution is to stop any supplement that contains biotin three days before your thyroid lab tests. To be safe, it is better to stop it before any lab test, as new research suggests that higher doses of biotin affect a whole range of blood tests. With deductibles as high as they are, it's probably best to avoid "lab do-overs." Be sure to read your supplement labels and make a list of the supplements with more than 1 mg of Biotin. Again, biotin is very helpful, and I use it regularly. Be sure to restrict its use around your blood draws.

Fasting & Morning Blood Draws

Many practitioners tell patients that fasting doesn't matter when testing the thyroid. Unfortunately, new research suggests that this isn't true for the TSH test. In one study, researchers found that eating before a draw can decrease TSH up to 26% compared to a fasting sample. I cannot help but wonder how many patients have had their medication reduced because of a post-meal TSH result! Fortunately, T4 and T3 labs do not appear to be affected by recent meals.

Recall that TSH naturally fluctuates during the day as it has its own circadian rhythm. Studies show that it is highest in the morning and lower later in the day. Since I already recommend fasting before getting drawn, it makes sense for most people to get drawn as early in the morning as possible. There are some people who, according to conventional medical models, would fit the diagnosis of hypothyroid unambiguously based on tests taken in the morning, but would be considered "borderline" by the same standards based on tests taken in the afternoon.

Of course, this wouldn't be as relevant if you were seeing a functional medicine practitioner who runs a complete thyroid panel, but for those of you currently stuck with TSH only, the time of day of your draw is a controllable variable that I recommend you monitor.

Take Your Thyroid Medication After Blood Tests

If you are taking thyroid medications, I recommend delaying your morning dose until after your blood draw. It's best to be safe because as your medication is absorbed into the bloodstream, it may produce inaccurate lab results. This pertains specifically to the thyroid hormone tests (T4 and T3) only.

TSH is not influenced by taking your morning dose medication. If your doctor is testing TSH only (which, to repeat, I think is too limited), it is okay to take your medication.

Taking T4-Only Medication

As an example, if you are prescribed Synthroid (or some other T4-only medication) and you took your medication at 6 am, and then went to the lab for an 8 am draw, you would be drawn at "dose peak" (highly concentrated in the blood) and your Free T4 would likely register as too high, likely leading to a reduction in medication strength. If, however, you were drawn at 7 am, only an hour after taking the Synthroid, the Free T4 would likely register as normal because the concentration of T4 would not yet have reached maximum concentration, which happens between two to four hours after taking the medication.

Taking T4/T3 Combo Medication

Medications that combine T4/T3 include all the natural desiccated thyroid, such as Armour thyroid, Nature-throid, NP thyroid, WP Thyroid, and the synthetic Thyrodol. Timing is even more critical when taking these medications because TSH, T3, and T4 are all affected, and all your thyroid lab results are likely to be inaccurate.

As soon as a T4/T3 medication is taken, the TSH immediately begins to drop and remains low for the next five hours. This is due to the fast-acting T3, which immediately enters tissues and starts activating the metabolism. The T3 labs will also change. They will be higher for four hours after taking the medication. Much like the T4-only medication example described above, the T4 lab results will be elevated up to four hours after taking the medication.

The bottom line: prevent inaccurate results by taking your medication immediately after your blood draw, not before.

The Functional Approach to Thyroid Lab Testing

Properly dosing thyroid medication requires the monitoring of three key aspects: blood tests, changes in symptoms, and exam findings (reflexes, temperature, pulse rate). In this section, the focus is on the labs that most accurately indicate thyroid status, plus other labs that provide a clear understanding of overall health. I'll review each lab test and explain what your lab test results mean. I'll also discuss lab tests that you will want to monitor in addition to the thyroid labs. Many of these additional tests relate to vitamins and minerals that help the thyroid function properly.

Thyroid Stimulating Hormone (TSH)

Thyroid Stimulating Hormone (TSH), also called thyrotropin, is a pituitary hormone that regulates the amount of thyroid hormone produced. The results of the TSH test can be confusing. Just remember that the results are the opposite of what the thyroid is doing. So, TSH is lower when there is too much thyroid hormone in circulation; TSH is higher when the body needs more thyroid hormone production.

TSH Ranges:
Standard Range: 0.5 – 5.5 mU/L
Optimal Range: 1.8 – 3.0 mU/L (Some experts say 1.0 to 2.0)

Free T4

This test measures the amount of free (unbound) T4 in the blood. Note that in this form T4 has limited activity. Sometimes this is ordered with TSH. Even so, it doesn't capture the entire thyroid picture. It does make up part of what I call the basic thyroid lab panel (along with TSH and Free T3). This lab value tends to fluctuate and is easily affected by thyroid medication (see section above).

Free T4 Ranges:
Standard Range: 0.7 – 1.8 ng/dL
Optimal Range: 1.0 – 1.5 ng/dL

Total T4

This lab is a measurement of all T4 hormone in circulation including T4 bound to a carrier protein and the unbound (free) T4 thyroid hormones. Many medications and supplements can alter this lab by affecting the hormone's ability to bind to proteins or to be absorbed. Estrogen, Lasix, iron, aspirin, steroids, and testosterone are just a few. If Total T4 and TSH are low, it's appropriate to suspect a low functioning pituitary.

Total T4 Ranges:
Standard Range: 4.5 – 12.0 ug/dL
Optimal Range: 6.0 – 12.0 ug/dL

Free T3

Free T3 is a measurement of the amount of unbound and active T3 thyroid hormone circulating in the blood stream. Unbound T3 can attach to a thyroid hormone receptor and activate cell metabolism immediately. It is one the most important indicators of both thyroid hormone conversion and thyroid hormone availability.

Total T3 Ranges:
Standard Range: 2.3 – 4.2 pg/mL
Optimal Range: 3.2 – 4.5 pg/mL

Total T3

Total T3 is the measurement of all T3 in the bloodstream including free T3 and reverse T3. In conventional medicine, this test is most commonly used to identify hyperthyroidism. In functional medicine circles, it is ordered to identify thyroid hormone conversion disorders. A selenium deficiency may lower total T3 test results.

Total T3 Ranges:
Standard Range: 60 – 181.0 ug/dL
Optimal Range: 100 – 180.0 ug/dL

Thyroid Antibodies

A thyroid antibody, or more accurately an "anti-thyroid antibody," is a protein created by your immune system that mistakenly recognizes your thyroid as a foreign invader and proceeds to attack parts of your thyroid with an enthusiasm normally reserved for the nastiest of bugs. There are many types of thyroid antibodies.

The two most common antibodies in Hashimoto's thyroiditis are thyroid peroxidase antibodies (TPOAb) and thyroglobulin antibodies (TGAb). The most commonly elevated of the two types of antibodies, anti-thyroid peroxidase antibodies, attack the thyroid peroxidase (TPO) enzyme that attaches iodine atoms to the building block of thyroid hormone called thyroglobulin. These antibodies can be elevated for years before the onset of hypothyroidism.

Anti-Thyroid Peroxidase Antibodies

TPO antibodies are strongly associated with iodine because increases in iodine in the thyroid trigger an increase in TPO enzyme production. About 85 to 90% of individuals with Hashimoto's will have elevated TPO antibodies. However it is rarely tested in conventional settings even when hypothyroid is present. More importantly, TPO antibody levels over 2000 increase the risk of other autoimmune diseases.

NOTE: Some labs have an upper limit to TPO antibodies. Quest Diagnostics has a cutoff of 900 with their standard thyroid antibody lab test. If your TPO antibody levels have been above 900 historically or if you are testing for the first time, I recommend getting the TPO antibody "Endpoint" test, which will give you the exact number.

Anti-TPO Antibody Ranges:
Standard Range: Less than 35.0 IU/mL (LabCorp) or 9.0 IU/mL (Quest and others).
Optimal Range: Undetectable.
Alarm Range: 2000.0+.

Thyroglobulin Antibodies

Slightly less common than TPO antibodies, thyroglobulin antibodies (TGAb) are found in 70% of cases of Hashimoto's thyroiditis. Thyroglobulin antibodies attack and destroy thyroglobulin, which can be thought of as the raw material from which thyroid hormone is created.

There is a strong association between high levels of thyroglobulin antibodies and thyroid cancer. Several studies have found that those over the age of 45 with Hashimoto's, thyroid nodules, and elevated TG antibodies (anything above "0") were at a greater risk of developing thyroid cancer. Elevated TPO anti-bodies alone don't appear to increase the risk, however.

Therefore, I automatically order an ultrasound for any patient with elevated thyroglobulin antibody levels who is over the age of 45. If you fit this picture, I would highly recommend getting an ultrasound just to be safe.

Thyroglobulin Antibody Ranges
Standard Range: Less than 1.0 IU/mL
Optimal Range: Undetectable

Reverse T3

I presented an in-depth look at reverse T3 (RT3) in Chapter 3 in which I explain that reverse T3 is an unusable form of T3 that blocks the thyroid hormone receptor sites on cells. Normally reverse T3 is created by the body to slow down the metabolism as a defense mechanism during injury, illness, and starvation. However, in our modern world, we more commonly see elevated Reverse T3 in chronic stress, low calorie "crash" diets, adrenal fatigue, nutrient deficiencies, and liver dysfunction.

I always recommend testing for reverse T3 as it can uncover the cause of low thyroid symptoms when more common labs (TSH, Free T4) come back normal.

Reverse T3 Ranges:
Standard Range: 7-25
Optimal Range: below 10

Free T3/Reverse T3 Ratio

This ratio is commonly used as a calculation to determine thyroid hormone conversion disorder trends. The consensus among functional medicine practitioners and thyroid advocates is that a ratio of 20 or more is ideal. However, a Free T3 that is above the upper range might make this ratio look healthier than it is. The best use of this ratio is when FT3 and RT3 are both within standard lab ranges.

Total T3/Reverse T3 Ratio

This ratio, used by the practitioners of the Institute of Functional Medicine, is for the same purpose - to detect conversion disorders. In this ratio, the ideal is 10 or higher. The Total T3/rT3 ratio and the Free T3/rT3 ratio can be used interchangeably. That said, I believe that the Total T3/rT3 ratio is a valuable tool for tracking the effectiveness of thyroid hormone conversion treatments over time and use it often in my practice.

Thyroid Blood Test Panels

As I have emphasized in this book, TSH-only lab testing misses a lot of variables, which can lead to misdiagnosis and inadequate treatment. We'll now review some additional thyroid lab panels that give you a more comprehensive thyroid picture.

The Comprehensive Thyroid Panel

This first panel is best when you are in investigation mode and haven't had much in the way of thyroid testing other than TSH or maybe Free T4. I will often order this panel for a new patient to give us a baseline of thyroid function. You'll notice that I include thyroid antibodies in this panel because of how common Hashimoto's thyroiditis is among those with thyroid conditions. This panel will consist of:

- TSH
- Free T4
- Total T4
- Free T3
- Total T3
- Thyroid Binding Globulin (or Sex Hormone Binding Globulin)
- Reverse T3
- Thyroid Peroxidase (TPO) Antibodies
- Thyroglobulin Antibodies
- TSH stimulating immunoglobulin (TSI) - *If symptoms of hyperthyroidism exist add to check for Graves' disease*

The results will give a complete picture of thyroid function. Nearly every possible thyroid dysfunction would show up in this lab series, which makes it ideal as an entry point for uncovering the underlying cause of thyroid problems or suspected thyroid conditions.

On thyroid panels available directly to consumers, you will encounter some variations, possibly Free Thyroxine Index or T3 Uptake. These are quite useful and provide a comprehensive overview.

After the first comprehensive thyroid panel, I'll often retest a patient about every four months, and I'll order the basic thyroid panel (see below) about six to eight weeks after the first test. Of course, this is assuming the tests come back relatively normal. I will retest labs that were abnormal in the first round of testing.

I typically check thyroid antibodies every six months if they are positive and yearly if they are negative. Since many factors can influence antibodies, they can fluctuate quite a bit. I tend to keep a close eye on TPO antibodies at 2000 or higher as the risk of other autoimmune diseases increases.

In case you need to order your own labs, I have included a lab resource section in the back of the book which provides information on labs that provide direct services to consumers.

The Basic Thyroid Panel

The basic thyroid panel is used to track the effectiveness of therapies over time. I consider this "bare bones" testing, but it's a suitable balance point between getting key information and keeping lab costs manageable.

- TSH
- Free T3
- Free T4
- Reverse T3

Thyroid Lab Patterns

Now that you have a basic understanding of thyroid lab tests, what these labs test for, and functional and conventional lab ranges, we can now put all of this information together and identify patterns.

Of course, I don't recommend trying to manage all of this on your own. This section is intended as a guide for you to consult regarding questions about your thyroid labs and before you see your health care practitioner so that you get the treatment plan that is right for you.

We're going to look at different types of lab patterns you might see on a comprehensive thyroid panel. This will give you an idea of what may be happening with your thyroid production and the effectiveness of your thyroid hormones.

Early Hashimoto's Thyroiditis

In the early stages of Hashimoto's the autoimmune attack on the thyroid is still developing. It has not yet damaged enough of the thyroid to disrupt thyroid hormone production to the extent that warrants a hypothyroidism diagnosis. Most of the thyroid lab results will be normal, though they may gradually edge toward lower thyroid hormone production. Thyroid antibodies are usually quite high.

- TSH: Normal or high normal
- T4 (total & free): Low or normal
- T3 (total & free): Low or normal
- Thyroid antibodies: High or very high
- Reverse T3: Varied

Primary Hypothyroidism/Mid-Stage Hashimoto's Thyroiditis

As you've learned in previous chapters, hypothyroidism is diagnosed because the thyroid isn't producing enough thyroid hormones to meet the needs of the body. Also recall that in most cases of hypothyroidism the depletion of hormone results from an autoimmune attack on the thyroid. Typically, medication is prescribed in conjunction with the diagnosis.

- TSH: High
- T4 (total & free): Low
- T3 (total & free): Low
- Thyroid antibodies: Very high in most cases
- Reverse T3: Varied, usually low

Pituitary Hypothyroidism (Secondary Hypothyroidism)

The pituitary doesn't produce enough TSH to address the body's need. This may be due to problems in the hypothalamus or in the pituitary itself.

- TSH: Low
- T4 (total & free): Low
- T3 (total & free): Low
- Thyroid antibodies: Varied, commonly none
- Reverse T3: Normal or low

Hypothalamus Hypothyroidism (Tertiary Hypothyroidism)

The hypothalamus doesn't accurately read thyroid hormone levels in the blood and cannot properly regulate thyroid production to address the body's needs.

- TSH: Low
- T4 (total & free): Low
- T3 (total & free): Low
- Thyroid antibodies: Varied, commonly none
- Reverse T3: Normal or low

Thyroid Hormone Conversion Syndrome/Selenium Deficiency

Thyroid hormone production in the thyroid is usually normal, but the peripheral conversion from T4 to T3 is reduced. T4 levels are normal or even high due to poor conversion. T3 levels are usually low, and conversion may be directed toward reverse T3. Selenium deficiency will commonly have the same lab pattern.

- TSH: Normal or slightly elevated
- T4 (total & free): Normal or high

- T3 (total & free): Low
- Thyroid antibodies: Varied
- Reverse T3: high, normal, or low

Iodine Deficiency

Less common since the introduction of iodized salt, however still present in some patients. If severe deficiency is present, labs typically resemble those of hypothyroidism. Mild deficiencies are more likely to show low T4 levels.

- TSH: Normal or high
- T4 (total & free): Low
- T3 (total & free): Low or normal
- Thyroid antibodies: Varied
- Reverse T3: Low

Hyperthyroidism/Graves' Disease

Labs indicate an overproduction of thyroid hormones. Thyroid antibodies are high. An additional lab test (TSI) is recommended to confirm hyperthyroidism. Reverse T3 is often high, which is beneficial in this case.

- TSH: Very low
- T4 (total & free): High
- T3 (total & free): High
- Thyroid antibodies: High - including TSH receptor stimulating antibodies (TSI)
- Reverse T3: Varied, usually high

Additional Labs Worth Considering

Other lab tests are important for the proper diagnosis of thyroid conditions. Most of these tests relate either to deficiencies that cause or exacerbate thyroid conditions or to deficiencies that must be addressed along with the thyroid to regain your health.

Vitamin D3

Vitamin D isn't actually a vitamin; it's a steroid, which means that your body can create it. Regardless, it is essential for our health and is commonly low due to sun avoidance, reduced intestinal absorption, and genetic factors. The use of sunscreen, while protective against skin cancer, has reduced our vitamin D production.

If you live in the Pacific Northwest as I do, the sun is a rare commodity for nearly half the year, and vitamin D levels plummet during this time. Many turn to vitamin D supplements which are a good idea, but those with digestive disorders are likely to have limited oral absorption. Genetic variations of vitamin D receptors can reduce cellular uptake of vitamin D into the cells themselves.

Recent research has found that the role of vitamin D extends well beyond bone health, with which it has long been associated. Vitamin D deficiency is widespread in those with low thyroid function. Research has discovered that it is especially important in thyroid health for several reasons.

First, vitamin D has a calming effect on the immune system when autoimmune conditions such as Hashimoto's and Grave's disease are present. Some researchers have suggested that vitamin D deficiency may be a cause of these conditions.

Second, vitamin D appears to have a role in regulating thyroid function. Research has found that low vitamin D levels (below 30 ng/mL) have an adverse effect on normal thyroid function. Test subjects with lower vitamin D have shown higher TSH levels than those with normal vitamin D levels.

Because vitamin D3 is a steroid, you can have toxic levels of vitamin D intake. It is recommended that you check your 25-Hydroxyvitamin D levels every three to four months if supplementing above 4000 IU daily. Supplemental vitamin D should be in D3 form and is best absorbed with other fat-soluble vitamins, especially vitamin K2.

Vitamin D3 Ranges:
Standard Range: 30-100 ng/mL

Optimal Range: 50-90 ng/mL

Selenium

We've discussed the importance of selenium in all aspects of thyroid function. It is safe to take up to 200 mcg daily. It is often helpful to check selenium levels to determine if a deficiency exists. Selenium toxicity is fairly rare.

Testing selenium is a bit tricky because two tests should be ordered. First, overall selenium levels can be determined with the "Selenium RBC" test. As RBC is an abbreviation for *red blood cell,* this test determines how much selenium has saturated into the red blood cell. This is more accurate than testing the amount of selenium floating in the bloodstream.

Selenium RBC Ranges:
Standard Range: 120-300 mcg/mL
Optimal Range: 225-300 mcg/mL

Even more important than the "Selenium RBC" test is the "Glutathione RBC" test. Once described as "the superhero of antioxidants" by Dr. Oz, glutathione plays a significant role in thyroid and cardiovascular health. It is one of the most effective detoxifying agents in your body and helps clean up the thyroid, especially in autoimmune thyroid conditions.

Selenium is a critical component in the formation of glutathione. So, by measuring your glutathione levels (again in the red blood cells), we can see how effective you are at reducing inflammation and free radical damage. It also indicates how well you use the selenium that you absorb. Most commercial labs offer this test.

Total Glutathione RBC Ranges:
Standard Range: 1,000 - 1,900 umol/L
Optimal Range: 1,400 - 1,900 umol/L

Iodine

Iodine is essential for normal thyroid function as it forms a crucial part of thyroid hormone. As mentioned above, with iodized salt now commonly available, the likelihood of iodine deficiency is assumed to be minimal. Still, while it is far less common to see iodine deficiency as we once did, I have encountered patients with low iodine.

No test is perfect, and iodine testing has its detractors. There are three schools of thought when it comes to iodine testing. The first recommends an iodine blood test, but this is least accurate of the tests available. The second supports an iodine challenge test with a 24-hour urine collection. The final approach is a simple random urine iodine test. As a simple baseline measurement, I prefer using the random urine iodine test, which most labs offer.

Iodine Urine (Random) Ranges:
Standard Range: 34 - 523 mcg/L
Optimal Range: 100-300 mcg/L

Zinc

Another important mineral for proper thyroid function is zinc. While iodine and selenium get most of the attention in the thyroid blogs, the unassuming zinc is essential in every step of the thyroid system.

It plays a vital role in thyroid regulation in the hypothalamus, hormone formation in the thyroid, thyroid hormone conversion, and thyroid receptor function. Since zinc is so critical to thyroid health, it makes sense to check your levels. I commonly find zinc deficiency in my patients. Like selenium, zinc is best measured in the red blood cells.

Zinc RBC Ranges:
Standard Range: 9.0 - 14.7 mg/L
Optimal Range: 13. - 14.7 mg/L

Magnesium

Magnesium is a mineral that gradually has been depleted in the soils of modern farms. As a result, magnesium is low in most people. It plays an important role in blood pressure and heart rhythm regulation, relaxes tight muscles, and helps with the production of T4 in the thyroid and the conversion from T4 to T3 in the organs. I recommend the Magnesium RBC test over the serum test as it is more accurate.

Magnesium RBC Ranges:
Standard Range: 4.0 - 6.4 mg/dL
Optimal Range: 6.0 - 6.5 mg/dL

Vitamin A

Vitamin A in the active form is called retinol. It plays an important role in thyroid function in two distinct ways. First, vitamin A activates the gene that regulates TSH production. Second, because it helps improve the sensitivity of the thyroid hormone receptors at the cellular level, it is an essential part of treating thyroid hormone resistance conditions.

Vitamin A is fat soluble, which means it can be toxic at high levels. For this reason, I recommend testing vitamin A to check for deficiencies and to monitor ongoing use of therapeutic daily intake.

Vitamin A Ranges:
Standard Range: 38-98 mcg/dL
Optimal Range: 68-98 mcg/dL

Comprehensive/Complete Iron Panel

Iron is another essential mineral used in many body functions. Most notably it is an essential component of the oxygen-carrying protein of the red blood cells called hemoglobin. About 65% of the iron in your body is found within the hemoglobin. A reduced capacity to circulate oxygen throughout the body is a serious health concern.

As previously stated in chapter 3, iron deficiency can decrease thyroid function in several ways. First, it can diminish the effectiveness of the hypothalamus and pituitary glands in regulating thyroid production. Next, iron is needed to make thyroid peroxidase enzyme required to produce thyroid hormone; an iron deficiency can reduce thyroid hormone production. Additionally, because iron is crucial to the thyroid hormone conversion process, a lack of iron can slow it down. Finally, as the thyroid hormone receptors within the cells are dependent on iron for proper functioning, low iron is associated with increased thyroid hormone resistance.

Four lab tests – serum iron, ferritin, iron saturation, and total iron-binding capacity (TIBC) – make up a complete iron panel. Serum iron measures the total iron circulating in your blood. Ferritin is the form of iron that is stored in your liver. Any iron that is not currently needed by the body is stored in the liver for later use. Transferrin is a carrier protein for iron that transports iron absorbed in your intestine throughout your body. The percentage of transferrin carrying iron is called Iron Saturation. Typically, about one-third of transferrin is transporting iron at any given time. The Total Iron Binding Capacity (TIBC) is an indirect measurement of the amount of transferrin in your body.

All of these tests except ferritin should be completed while fasting. No iron supplements should be taken for 5 days prior to testing. The ranges for these labs are as follows:

Serum Iron Ranges:
Standard Range: 40.0 - 160.0 ug/dL
Optimal Range: 85.0 - 130.0 ug/dL

Ferritin Ranges:
Standard Range: 10.0 - 232.0 ng/mL
Optimal Range: 50.0 - 70.0 ng/mL

Iron/Transferrin Saturation Ranges:
Standard Range: 15 - 50%
Optimal Range: 35 - 38%

<u>Total Iron Binding Capacity (TIBC) Ranges:</u>
Standard Range: 250.0 - 425.0 ug/dL
Optimal Range: 250.0 - 350.0 ug/dL

The Role of Thyroid Ultrasound

Conventional medicine uses thyroid ultrasound to identify the type of nodules that are found during a thyroid exam. Most thyroid nodules are benign, but some can indicate thyroid cancer or pre-cancer, both of which require medical intervention.

Thyroid ultrasound is non-invasive and painless, and a radiologist will review the ultrasound images for any changes to the thyroid size, tissue, and blood flow. I am a big fan of thyroid ultrasound tests as they help track changes in the thyroid, which is especially important with conditions such as Hashimoto's thyroiditis, hyperthyroidism (Graves' disease), and thyroid cancer.

Establishing a Thyroid Baseline

I use thyroid ultrasound imaging a bit differently than my conventional counterparts, however. Most conventional healthcare practitioners believe that a thyroid ultrasound should be limited to those patients who have palpable thyroid nodules.

For most of my patients, I encourage getting a baseline ultrasound as a screening tool if the thyroid is not able to produce thyroid hormones on its own. Here's my reasoning: the development of thyroid nodules is more likely in those with autoimmune thyroiditis. Some of these thyroid nodules can become cancerous.

By getting this baseline thyroid ultrasound, I can determine the current health of the thyroid tissue, and with further ultrasounds, I can track changes to the thyroid over time and take action early if a suspicious nodule appears.

Confirming and Tracking Autoimmune Thyroid Disease

As mentioned in this and other chapters, Hashimoto's thyroiditis is the most common form of hypothyroidism in the industrialized world. For 85 to 90% of those with Hashimoto's, the thyroid antibodies test will provide a rough indication of the level of tissue destruction within the thyroid. The other 10 to 15% will never have thyroid antibodies but will have thyroid tissue destruction all the same.

For this reason, it makes sense to confirm an autoimmune process for those who don't have measurable thyroid antibodies. Based on my clinical experience, I find that about 10% of my hypothyroid patients with normal antibodies will have signs of tissue destruction with ultrasound testing. The other 5% experience thyroid hormone conversion or resistance due to other factors.

The level of thyroid antibodies correlates somewhat with the rate of tissue destruction. Using thyroid ultrasound gives you a clear indication of the extent of thyroid tissue damage. As a rule, I order thyroid ultrasound imaging every two years for anyone who has TPO antibodies around 1000 and yearly for those with TPO antibodies over 2000.

Making Sure You Don't Have Thyroid Cancer

Conventional medicine widely recognizes the increased risk of thyroid cancer among those with Hashimoto's thyroiditis. The actual risk comes from having elevated thyroglobulin antibodies as mentioned earlier in this chapter. The risk increases when nodules are present in people over the age of 45.

ThyroFlex Testing:

The fundamental issue with correcting thyroid problems is determining how well thyroid hormones are being used in the cells. All the blood tests available today only offer a partial glimpse into thyroid function. It is for this reason that a comprehensive thyroid panel is used. Each lab test is a puzzle piece.

Unfortunately, when they are all put together, they still don't complete the puzzle entirely, as many patients assume. There are very few lab tests that give insight into how well thyroid hormone is activating metabolism at the cellular level. To determine thyroid function, savvy providers look for clues in symptoms, visual signs observed during examination, basal body temperature, and Achilles heel reflex testing.

All of these indicators are somewhat reliable, but I have discovered a much more accurate testing method called the ThyroFlex test. It was created by Daryl Turner, Ph.D. and the late Konrad Kail, ND, and it is based on the deep tendon reflex test used by doctors before thyroid labs were available. ThyroFlex measures the reflex time of the forearm, which is then analyzed on a laptop. This offers a graphical representation of thyroid function.

Having used this test, I find it to be invaluable in confirming thyroid disorders in those with normal lab results but classic symptoms of low thyroid function. Furthermore, I can retest with the Thyroflex in my office and get instant feedback on treatment progress.

Chapter Highlights

- Thyroid hormone tests are sensitive to fasting, thyroid medication, and the supplement biotin. Therefore, it's best to get drawn in the early morning while fasting, waiting to take any thyroid medication until after the blood test. Avoid biotin intake for 72 hours.

- Comprehensive thyroid testing provides a fairly complete picture of your thyroid function. I recommend using the optimal lab values found in this chapter to determine how well your thyroid system is working.

- Additional labs may be needed to assess nutrient status and determine if anemias are present.

- Thyroid ultrasound is an inexpensive and effective means of detecting pathological changes in the thyroid gland.

- ThyroFlex testing is an in-office procedure that tests your reflexes to determine how well T3 thyroid hormone is entering the cells. Use in conjunction with comprehensive thyroid testing, a complete picture of thyroid health and function immerges.

CHAPTER 8

Optimizing Thyroid Medications

An Introduction and Brief History of Thyroid Medication

AS WE ENTER THIS CHAPTER, I'd like to address some important questions that I am commonly asked in my clinical practice. "Do I need thyroid medication?" "If so, is it for the rest of my life?" "What thyroid medication will work best for me?" "Which is better, synthetic or natural thyroid medication?" "Are there alternatives to medication?"

In this chapter, each of these questions will be answered in detail. Additionally, we will focus on the pros and cons of the different types of thyroid medication. I will explain how the fillers in medication can cause problems for some users, help you determine how you could be affected, and explore alternative medication options.

The history of treating thyroid disorders can be traced back thousands of years. Ancient murals, paintings, and sculptures show people with swollen thyroid glands (goiters). Descriptions of this condition have been found in writings going back as far as

2700 BC. It appears that iodine deficiency caused this massive grapefruit-sized swelling of the thyroid.

There is evidence that Chinese, Indian Ayurvedic, and Greek physicians were aware of and attempted to treat these thyroid conditions. The use of seaweed and other herbs was found to be helpful, which makes sense because seaweed is very high in iodine. There are indications that animal thyroid tissues may have been used, but it doesn't seem to have been a common practice.

The use of extracted animal thyroid in treating hypothyroidism, which gained popularity in the 1890s, was a watershed advancement. In 1955, treatment changed again when Synthroid was developed by Abbott Laboratories. It was the first synthetic T4 medication brought to market. Many generic brands entered the market shortly thereafter. By the 1980s the use of T4-only medication became the most common way to treat hypothyroidism. As a therapy, it works for many but certainly not all.

Do You Need Thyroid Medication?

This is a very important question that has several answers. Most are prescribed T4 thyroid medication due to high TSH lab levels, indicating that the thyroid isn't making thyroid hormone as directed by the pituitary. For all intents and purposes, this approach is conventional medicine's only therapeutic option. Usually, those on T4 medication are told that they will be taking the medication for the rest of their lives.

For some, unfortunately, this is true, especially for those whose thyroid glands have been damaged beyond their ability to produce enough thyroid hormone to meet the body's needs. A textbook example of this would be late-stage Hashimoto's thyroid disease, in which scar tissue has replaced most of the thyroid-producing cells. Similarly, those with either partial or complete thyroid gland removal will need additional thyroid hormone through medication for the rest of their lives.

However, there are situations in which thyroid hormone deficiency can be reversed without the need for thyroid medication by taking herbs, vitamins, and minerals. Because the topic of nutrition isn't a significant part of the conventional medical model, it has been ridiculed and ignored as a therapeutic option.

Nonetheless, holistic and functional medicine practitioners have found nutrients to be essential for addressing overall thyroid dysfunction, whether the problem is within the thyroid or occurs in the peripheral tissues.

Most people with thyroid disorders have one or more nutrient deficiencies. When these deficiencies are corrected, thyroid function greatly improves. This includes conditions such as autoimmune thyroid disorders in which an overactive immune system destroys the thyroid cells. Admittedly, it takes concerted effort to reverse the autoimmune process in these cases, but it is possible.

As a rule, I believe that thyroid medication should be regarded as a temporary solution until the body can be recalibrated to ensure the thyroid hormone works optimally in the body again. It is best to think of thyroid medication as a "triage medicine," a medication that is used until the underlying cause of the thyroid disorder is fixed. I never recommend anyone stop thyroid medication without a gradual reduction in dose under careful medical supervision.

Next, we will look at the individual medications, treatment approaches, and alternatives for those with allergies and sensitivities.

Which Medications Work Best?

For many of my patients, the T4-only medication fails to ease or eliminate the thyroid symptoms they are experiencing. It is estimated that about 70% of those prescribed T4-only therapy experience adequate relief from hypothyroid symptoms. In my experience, I believe the percentage of symptom relief is closer to 60%.

Patients who find their way to my clinic are usually within the 40% of those with low thyroid function who have T3 thyroid hormone problems. Most of these patients have healthcare practitioners who either refuse to use T4/T3 combo medications or dismiss their remaining thyroid symptoms as deriving from other conditions.

Problems with Inactive Ingredients (aka Fillers)

One of the issues with these commercially produced medications, whether it is T4 or T3 medication, is the fillers that make up the base of the tablets. Only a small portion of the pill is actual thyroid hormone; the rest consists of binders, artificial food dyes, and chemicals that help the tablet function properly. Any number of these filler agents may elicit an allergic reaction or affect absorption in the intestines.

One type of problematic filler is gluten-based starch. Not all starches are gluten-based, but as of the writing of this book, there are no FDA rules about labeling medications as gluten-free. This means that pharmaceutical companies can switch the source of fillers from potato-based starch to a gluten-derived starch without notice.

I have many patients with Celiac disease, a severe autoimmune based gluten allergy (see chapter 9). These individuals cannot tolerate gluten in any amount. About half of the human population is affected. The rates are lower in Caucasians and much higher in those of African, Asian, and Jewish descent. There are efforts to require labels indicating a gluten-free status on all prescription and over-the-counter medications.

For those of you who have celiac disease, gluten sensitivity, or Hashimoto's hypothyroidism, it is crucial to consult with your practitioner and pharmacist and explore online resources. One my favorite sites is www.glutenfreedrugs.com, which is run and updated continuously by a clinical pharmacist. It is a valuable resource for anyone with gluten sensitivities or allergies. In my practice, I always write a note to the pharmacist indicating that they should only dispense gluten-free medication.

Keep in mind that lactose (milk sugar), often used in the form of lactose monohydrate, can trigger symptoms in those with celiac disease and may limit medication absorption in those with lactose intolerance. For those with celiac disease, strict avoidance is recommended. Lactose intolerant patients may need to increase their thyroid medication dose to compensate for any decrease in absorption.

Finally, those who are sensitive to artificial food coloring should be aware that many of the thyroid medications contain one or more food dyes. ADD/ADHD tendencies are usually aggravated by consuming artificial food coloring. I highly recommend limiting your intake of these food dyes.

Synthetic vs. Natural Desiccated Thyroid (NDT)?

To some degree this is a matter of preference; either can be useful when used correctly. As mentioned above, the fillers can be problematic for some, which will influence medication choices. Those following a plant-based, kosher, or halal diet may wish to avoid medications that include pork-derived thyroid tissue.

Most conventional practitioners discourage the use of desiccated thyroid. The most common reason is the four-parts-T4-to-one-part-T3 ratio found in NDT. This ratio is normal for pigs, but humans have a 14:1 ratio of T4 to T3. The detractors argue that the T3 in the medication is too much for the human body.

I disagree. Most tolerate NDT well, provided the dose meets their needs. There are concerns about the pork origin of NDT and the risk of contracting swine flu, but they are overstated. Such risk is extremely low as viruses don't survive the purification process for NDT.

Most of my patients feel better taking a medication containing a combination of T4 and T3. Natural desiccated thyroid is a convenient and inexpensive choice. That said, you can expect to encounter resistance from most conventional practitioners. I recommend seeking out a naturopathic or functional medicine physician in your area as they are more likely to prescribe NDT.

Synthetic T4 Medication - Levothyroxine

Levothyroxine is the pharmaceutical name for the T4-only medication. The four big brand names are Levoxyl, Unithroid, Levotroid, and Synthroid. These brand names, along with generic forms of levothyroxine, all contain the same amount of T4. What makes them different is the fillers used. This is an important aspect to consider for those with moderate to severe food allergies, especially for those with Celiac disease.

Synthroid was the first synthetic T4 medication commercially available beginning in the late 1950's. It quickly became the medication of choice for most medical practitioners in the United States and the UK, replacing the natural desiccated thyroid hormone commonly used at the time. This change was in part due to the aggressive marketing campaign by Abbott to convince doctors that Synthroid was the only form of thyroid medication that could be trusted be pure and to have a consistent amount of medication.

Since that time, many generic forms of levothyroxine have become available alongside the brand names listed above. The fillers used in levothyroxine can include gluten-based starch. This is common, and I believe it is worth paying attention to if you have Hashimoto's thyroiditis or gluten sensitivity.

The following levothyroxine medications have been confirmed as gluten-free:

- Synthroid
- Levoxyl
- Certain Levothyroxine Generics (Sigma pharma, Mylan, Lannett, and Sandoz brands)

Tirosint

Tirosint is the purest form of T4 medication as it only contains four ingredients, the levothyroxine medication and three fillers (gelatin, glycerin, and water). Even the most allergic of individuals tolerate Tirosint. This Swiss made medication is manufactured in a facility free of allergens and contaminants. Learn more at their website: www.tirosint.com.

I have prescribed this medication for several years and no patient has encountered problems with it. The downside is the price, which averages $150/month. Unfortunately, many medical insurance companies are resistant to covering this medication instead of generic levothyroxine.

Synthetic T4/T3 Medication

Liotrix (Thyrolar)

Liotrix is a synthetic medication containing both T4 and T3 medication in the same 4:1 ratio found in the natural desiccated thyroid (NDT) hormone extracted from pork thyroid. This is a suitable option for those unable to use NDT. The filler agents contain artificial coloring, lactose, and cornstarch.

Thyrolar is the only form of Liotrix available in the U.S. but has been unavailable due to shortages at the time of writing this book. The FDA indicates that this medication will likely become available in late 2018.

Synthetic T3 Medication

Liothyronine is the pharmaceutical name of synthetic T3, first synthesized in 1926, but not commercially available until 1956.

Liothyronine is fast acting with 95% of the medication absorbed within 4 hours. Synthetic T3 is biologically active and acts immediately on the tissues of the body, bypassing the thyroid hormone conversion enzymes. This is advantageous for those who have problems with thyroid hormone conversion or thyroid hormone resistance due to genetics, nutrient deficiency, and inflammation. Liothyronine is available in 5 mcg, 25 mcg, and 50 mcg tablets.

Liothyronine is safe when used correctly but be aware that you are likely to experience resistance from many practitioners. The only side effects occur when the dosage is too high. Symptoms of excessive T3 intake include accelerated pulse, headaches, tremors, nervousness, trouble sleeping, and sensitivity to heat.

You are more likely to experience side effects if you have Adrenal Fatigue syndrome or another adrenal gland disorder. People with diabetes need to watch their blood sugar carefully as insulin and blood sugar levels may fluctuate due to the liothyronine. Such fluctuation may require adjusting diabetic medications. Finally, T3 medication is known to interact with over 200 medications including depression and anxiety medications, birth control pills, diabetes medications, and several vitamins and minerals. Be sure to review with your provider before using liothyronine.

Cytomel

Manufactured by Pfizer and first available in 1956, Cytomel is the brand name of liothyronine. There have been problems with Cytomel's filler agents, which have rotated among gluten, potato, and cornstarch, causing reactions in those with gluten sensitivities.

As of 2016, they have stopped using gluten and potato starches and have switched to cornstarch exclusively. Still, they do not do any post-production testing for gluten, so cross-contamination is possible. For this reason, I prefer using generic forms of liothyronine; some of these brands are confirmed to be gluten-free.

Liothyronine

There are many manufacturers of generic liothyronine. Because all generic forms contain the same amount of T3, attention should be directed toward the inactive ingredients to determine which filler agents could be problematic for sensitive individuals. Three manufacturers of liothyronine (Mylan, Paddock, and Sigma-pharm) are recommended over all others because they do not use gluten in their fillers.

Of these three, only Mylan is tested to ensure gluten-free status. The other two companies do not use gluten in their fillers but do not perform any post-production tests either. I've prescribed all three medications, and my gluten sensitive patients have done well with them.

Slow-Release T3

Because T3 is so fast acting, the use of a slow-release T3 (SRT3) has become more popular with some practitioners, especially those using the Wilson Temperature Syndrome approach. This has a few advantages over the standard T3 medication. First, SRT3 eliminates the side effects of T3 – feeling jittery, nervous, and having tremors – which is especially helpful for those with adrenal conditions. Second, there is a constant trickle of T3 released into the bloodstream over 12 hours, ensuring a consistent presence of T3 in the body. Finally, this method is more convenient for patients as there are fewer pills to take during the day.

Slow-release T3 is only available through compounding pharmacies who will custom-make your medication. An advantage to this approach is greater control of the fillers used. During the production process, the pharmacist creates multiple layers of the liothyronine, which are then covered by a filler shell. As the shell layer breaks down, more T3 is absorbed into the bloodstream. Because slow-release T3 is more slowly absorbed, each tablet must contain two and a half times the amount of T3 as a standard T3 dose/tablet.

Depending on your provider's approach, you would take a single tablet in the morning or one every 12 hours (typically 6 am and 6 pm). Some practitioners criticize this approach because it bypasses the body's natural thyroid hormone rhythm. However, this is true of thyroid medication in general. Overall, most people taking SRT3 are delighted with the results and find the medicine easy to take with very few of the side effects associated with regular liothyronine.

Natural Desiccated Thyroid (T4/T3)

The use of thyroid hormone replacement can be traced back to the late 19th century when the use of organotherapy – the ingestion of animal endocrine glands to address endocrine disorders in humans – became popular. The use of thyroid gland to treat hypothyroidism quickly became the standard of care in the 1890 and remains somewhat popular in alternative medicine circles. However, the inconsistency of the amount of thyroid hormone found in the raw thyroid extract was a significant problem as one batch would have too much thyroid and another too little.

Before long, the process of extracting the thyroid hormone from the pig thyroid became routinized, and there emerged several large pharmaceutical manufacturers of desiccated thyroid hormone, which was supplied to pharmacists who then created medications locally for patients. However, there were still some inconsistencies with the amount of thyroid hormone found in the tablets. In part, this was because T3 wasn't discovered until 1952. Another complicating factor was that the primary measurement was the amount of iodine alone.

Manufacturers that have continued to operate from the beginning include the pharmaceutical branch of the Armour meatpacking company, which still produces Armour thyroid. Today there are several producers of desiccated thyroid hormone, and they all use pig thyroid. There are a few raw thyroid extracts sourced from beef thyroid, all of which are sold over-the-counter as supplements. The companies do not measure the amount of T4 to T3 in the tablets produced, so there is no guarantee of consistent dosage.

Is NDT Safe to Use with Hashimoto's Thyroiditis?

There are reports that use of desiccated thyroid exacerbates the antibodies of Hashimoto's. Such an adverse reaction is associated with the introduction of additional TPO enzymes and thyroglobulin, which triggers a heightened autoimmune response.

In my clinical experience, I have never seen anyone's antibodies increase from taking NDT. In fact, I have seen the opposite: antibodies dropping with the use of NDT.

Overall, desiccated thyroid is safe to use as it is purified, processed, and standardized to contain an exact amount of T4 and T3 with every dose. Additionally, NDT includes T2, T1, and calcitonin, though they are not measured or standardized.

The Different Brands of NDT

There are four major brands of natural desiccated thyroid, Armour, NP-thyroid, Nature-throid, and WP-thyroid. All are made from pork thyroid tissue and share a 4:1 thyroid hormone ratio among the brands.

Most tablets will come in several different strengths with "1 grain" commonly used, which equals 60 or 65 mg. Among the brands, 1 grain of NDT will consistently contain 38 mcg of T4 and 9 mcg of T3, the rest of the tablet is filler. The primary difference between the brands is the filler agents used.

Awareness of the different fillers used is important, especially if you have allergies, since some NDT may contain gluten, lactose, corn, soy or potato extracts.

For example, the makers of Armour thyroid don't use gluten byproducts as a filler, but they also don't perform any final analy-

Dr. Shawn Soszka

sis to guarantee gluten-free status. Their fillers are corn-, potato-, and soy-free.

Compare this to Nature-throid, which is gluten-free, but contains a small amount of lactose. There are several other lesser known brands to choose from, but my preference is either Nature-throid or WP-thyroid both made by RLC labs.

Controlling Fillers
Compounded Thyroid Medication

Throughout this chapter, I've discussed the different types of thyroid medication commercially available. The inactive ingredient fillers used in these medications can be problematic for those who are sensitive, especially to gluten, corn, and lactose. If you are one of these people, I highly recommend exploring compounded medication.

Compounding pharmacies custom-make your medication, carefully avoiding the filler agents containing allergenic ingredients. The cost is higher than commercially produced drugs, but I believe the benefits and peace of mind are worth it.

Keep in mind that problematic fillers may be in other medications you may be taking. If you suspect this is the case, I recommend carefully reviewing the lists of medications found on www.glutenfreedrugs.com. Be sure to check the "new list" link as it contains more information about fillers made from gluten, corn, soy, lactose, and potato.

If you wish to learn more about the compounded medications or to find a compounding pharmacy I recommend the Professional Compounding Centers of America (www.pccarx.com) which is a professional association of over 4000 pharmacies in the United States. They provide a directory of U.S. compounding pharmacies searchable by city, state, and zip code.

For readers outside of the United States, the International Academy of Compounding Pharmacists (www.iacprx.org) provides an <u>international directory</u> with pharmacies in Canada, the UK, Australia, and a few countries in Central America, Europe, and Asia. This information is also available in the Resources Appendix at the end of the book.

Chapter Highlights

- Levothyroxine (T4-only) medication often fails to completely address the symptoms of hypothyroid and low thyroid function. Talk to your pharmacist about your levothyroxine prescription to make sure it is gluten-free.

- Tirosint is an extremely pure form of levothyroxine, a highly beneficial option for those who are highly sensitive to fillers.

- Liothyronine (T3-only) medication is a fast-acting medication. It is often used in addition to levothyroxine but can be used by itself. In many low thyroid situations, such as thyroid hormone conversion disorders and thyroid hormone resistance, T3 is an important component to restoring proper function.

- Slow-Release T3 (SRT3) is specially formulated liothyronine designed to "trickle" a consistent amount of T3 into the bloodstream over a 12-hour period. This method eliminates symptoms in highly sensitive individuals. A compounding pharmacist must make SRT3.

- Combination T4/T3 medications often help improve and stabilize low thyroid symptoms. Natural desiccated thyroid (NDT) is extracted from pig thyroid gland and has a standardized 4:1 dose of T4 and T3.. I recommend Nature-throid and WP-thyroid by RLC labs.

- Filler agents in medications can contain ingredients made from potentially allergenic substances, such as wheat, corn, soy, and potato.

- Those reactive to one or more allergens can benefit from having medications custom-made through compounding pharmacies. These specialized pharmacists can work with you to make a medication that works best for your body.

CHAPTER 9

The Best Thyroid Diet

Core Principles of a Healthy Eating Plan

THERE IS A LOT OF CONFLICTING INFORMATION online about which diet is best for people with thyroid disorders. In this chapter, I review some of the popular diets and discuss their pro and cons in regard to improving thyroid function.

Before we look at the diets, it is essential to see the standard American diet (SAD) for what it is: high in carbohydrates, full of bad fat, pro-inflammatory, with very little nutrients. Our way of eating is destroying our health like never before.

Today we have access to more food than at any point in history, yet we still fail to get the recommended daily allowance (RDA) of vitamins and minerals from our daily intake. The situation looks even worse when you consider that the RDA guidelines consist of the bare minimum, only what is needed to keep diseases at bay. It doesn't come close to optimizing your health. The nutrients we need are available to us. We merely need to change our approach to eating and seek out foods that contain what we need.

Fortunately, diet is one of the health variables that we can control because, of course, we choose what we put in our bodies.

Therefore, I recommend making the diet changes outlined in this chapter to help you reboot your body and provide it with the nutrients it needs to begin the healing process. Most readers will have a common sense understanding of healthy versus unhealthy foods, so we'll start there and build a logical diet framework.

A Basic Plan for Healthy Eating

A vital component of a healthy diet is emphasizing healing, anti-inflammatory foods and eliminating inflammation-causing, allergenic foods. First, let us discuss anti-inflammatory foods.

1. Organic Vegetables and Fruits
2. Organic Grass-Fed/Finished Meats
3. Organic, Free-Range Chicken and High Omega-3 Eggs
4. Wild Caught Fish
5. Limited Gluten-Free Whole Grains
6. Limited Organic Dairy (A2 Origin, Goat, or Sheep)
7. Legumes

In addition, to which foods to eat, I want to emphasize the importance of getting enough caloric intake. Based on my clinical experience, I have found a segment of those with low thyroid function who try to restrict calories as means of losing weight.

Portion control is fine, but those who significantly reduce calorie intake (often under 800 calories per day), such as those on the HCG diet, ketogenic diet, or other highly restrictive diets, will slow down thyroid function even further. It is far more important to eat a healthy, low-inflammatory diet than to try to restrict calories.

Vegetables and Fruits

Plenty of vegetables and a moderate amount of fruit should be the cornerstone of your new diet. This is by far one of the easiest and most important lifestyle changes you can make for improving your health. There is plenty of research that shows a diet rich in vegetables helps slow the aging process. Vegetables can also lower the risk of heart disease, cancer, and dementia. Plants are high in omega-3 fats and vitamins B and C, all of which improve mood and stress resiliency. Green leafy vegetables such as Swiss chard, kale, and spinach have high amounts of magnesium that can help reduce high blood pressure. The fiber in vegetables helps gut motility operate correctly.

About 40-50% of your lunch and dinner plate should be vegetables. Organic and GMO-free vegetables are the best choice. See the section below about organic exceptions if you are on a budget.

Try to eat vegetables from all colors of the rainbow to get more antioxidants. Vegetables are best prepared when steamed or lightly stir-fried. Raw vegetables are also a healthy choice BUT beware of raw cruciferous vegetables (see the section below) as they can slow your thyroid function.

There are a couple of vegetables I recommend eliminating: potatoes and corn. Both have little fiber, can raise the blood sugar quickly, and may be inflammatory (see below).

Cruciferous Vegetables: Facts and Myths

For many years patients have asked me if eating cruciferous vegetables such as kale, broccoli, and collard greens were bad for thyroid function. This idea stems from older nutritional books that identified these cruciferous vegetables as causing thyroid goiters and hypothyroidism, in addition to a few studies that found some correlation between the two.

Before we go any further, I want to identify the commonly consumed cruciferous vegetables, which include Brussel sprouts, swiss chard, arugula, bok choy, broccoli, cauliflower, kale, cabbage, collard greens, mustard greens, radishes, kohlrabi, and soy.

One study found that a high intake of these vegetables triggers hypothyroidism in lab animals. Cruciferous vegetables contain a sulfur-based chemical called glucosinolates, which can affect those with extreme iodine deficiency, especially when eaten raw. Concerns subsided when another study found that eating 5 oz of brussels sprouts a day for four weeks didn't affect the thyroid whatsoever. Overall, the bulk of research indicates that cruciferous vegetables are safe to eat, especially when cooked.

Since the green leafy vegetables that make up most of the cruciferous family are full of vitamins and minerals, I highly recommend eating them, but cooked rather than raw as to minimize any risk. Increased vegetable intake is vital to the recovery of your health. The cruciferous group of vegetables is an excellent source of nutrients and the fiber that your intestinal bacteria needs to optimize your health.

Nightshade Vegetables

There is research that indicates that the nightshade family of vegetables can cause inflammation in the intestines and the joints. Not everyone will be reactive to these foods, but anyone with a thyroid problem should seriously consider this possibility.

Nightshades include potatoes, tomatoes, eggplant, goji berries, chilies, and bell peppers. They contain alkaloids (glycoalkaloids and steroid alkaloids) that have been shown to cause inflammation and can trigger leaky gut in those with poor digestion, celiac disease, and those genetically predisposed to inflammatory bowel disease. Reactions are often more severe in non-organic nightshade foods, especially potatoes and tomatoes.

Additionally, nightshades are associated with muscle aches and joint inflammation, which causes pain and stiffness. This may be due to the increased risk of intestinal inflammation. In both instances, intestinal permeability and increased food sensitivities/allergies are commonly seen.

Since there is a relationship between thyroid disorders and the digestive tract, I think it is a good idea for those with low thyroid function to temporarily remove nightshade vegetables from your diet.

Typically, a 30-day removal of nightshades is recommended followed by a careful reintroduction as a trial to determine reactivity. After the 30 days, begin by adding a small amount (about one tablespoon) of a single nightshade vegetable (potato or tomato, for instance) for three consecutive dinners. If no noticeable reaction occurs, wait a day, and then add the next nightshade using this same approach. Continue this until all the nightshade vegetables have been successfully reintroduced. If you don't notice any reactions, then you can add them back into your diet. However, if you do have any reaction, stop the reintroduction, and continue to avoid any nightshades for, at least, another week and try again. If a reaction occurs a second time, it is best to avoid that vegetable.

Not everyone will react to nightshade vegetables. Some will react to one or two of the nightshades. Others can't tolerate nightshades at all and should avoid them entirely. Those of you who find yourself reacting to nightshades need to read labels carefully. Pay particular attention to potato starch, which is commonly found in packaged foods.

Fruit

Fruit is full of antioxidants, especially berries. I recommend organic fruit since so many contain pesticide residues. Studies have found that organic fruits have more nutrients compared to their conventionally grown counterparts.

The sugar content of fruit can be a concern as fruit can be high in fructose. When accompanied by fiber this sugar absorbs slowly into the bloodstream. In other forms, such as fruit juice, fructose enters the bloodstream quickly where it is transported to the liver for conversion to glucose. Whereas fructose must be converted first, glucose is usable by every cell in the body.

A healthy liver is able to convert a small amount of fructose without any difficulties, but fruit high in fructose and little fiber can overwhelm the liver. In such cases, fructose is converted to fat stored in the liver, which can lead to elevated cholesterol and triglycerides. Likewise, excessive fructose can lead to insulin resistance, obesity, and even gout attacks!

Don't get me wrong, fruit is a rich source of vitamins, but we need to be aware of the sugar content. In most cases, raw fruit have a good fiber-to-sugar ratio. Avocados, olives, lemons, and most berries have some of the best fiber-to-sugar ratios.

On the opposite side of the spectrum, grapes and strawberries are high in fructose and low in fiber. Consuming 20 grapes has nearly the same sugar content as drinking a can of Coca-Cola. Other fruit sources high in sugar are dried fruits, canned fruits, and fruit juice. As a rule, fruit juice should be limited to about 8 to 12 ounces per week, if not eliminated entirely.

Fiber & Microbiome

Our large intestine is host to trillions of microbes, entire metropolises of bacteria, fungi, viruses, and other microbial life forms, all competing for resources. Collectively referred to as the microbiome, these microorganisms have an impact on our health that is difficult to overstate. While there is a benefit in using probiotics to strengthen healthy bacterial strains, research has found that fiber is more effective at feeding the good bacteria already in our gut.

Fiber has long been associated with improving bowel movement, and its role is even more significant than previously realized. Studies find that fiber is the fuel source of the healthy bacteria, while yeast and harmful bacteria prefer our high sugar intake. One such study found that increased fiber shifted the microbiome from bacterial species associated with obesity to those known to promote a leaner body type. Additionally, these fiber-loving microbes produce vitamins and play an important role in the conversion of T4 into the active thyroid hormone T3.

One of my biggest complaints about the popularity of "low carb diets" is the lack of fiber that so often accompanies these approaches. We're already starved of fiber in the Western world, consuming about 15 grams per day, a trifle compared to the 150 grams that our Neolithic ancestors consumed. There is plenty of research that shows that our lower fiber intake puts our microbiome at risk. Even friendly bacteria can turn on us in desperation when they starve.

The Benefits of Organic Produce

Buying organic produce is another way to improve your health. Many of the pesticides used in modern farming are linked to dozens of health problems, including certain cancers, symptoms of ADHD, autism, and Parkinson's.

Moreover, pesticides can impair the thyroid, digestion, and other organ systems. This is especially relevant today since so much of our produce is imported from places where pesticide laws are laxer. Even DDT, a pesticide banned in the US for years, has been detected in imported food.

While there are many health advantages to eating organic, it can be a bit pricey! The good news is that there is an excellent organization called the Environmental Working Group, (www.ewg.org) which regularly tests produce for pesticide residue. It provides an annual report called the "Dirty Dozen, Clean 15." In it, you will find the 12 (or more) fruits and vegetables that are most harmful when conventionally produced. Likewise, they list the 15 produce items least affected by pesticides. This guide is especially handy if you want to eat healthily and are watching your food budget.

This list should not discourage you from eating fruits and vegetables, but it should make you wary of current farming practices.

The use of chemicals to kill weeds, microbes, and insects has some unwelcome side effects. It can sap nutrients from the soil and kill helpful microbes.

Topping the 2017 dirty dozen report are strawberries, which can contain up to 20 different pesticide residues. Spinach comes in second with the highest pesticide-per-weight ratio on the list. DDT and known neurotoxins are among the residues found in spinach samples tested. Every item on this list tested positive for, at least, one pesticide.

EWG also has a phone app to make your smart shopping much more manageable. I highly recommend it. The 2018 Dirty Dozen list has not been released as of the publication of this book. Kindle readers can expect this section to be updated as new information becomes available.

2017 Dirty Dozen List
1. Strawberry
2. Spinach
3. Nectarines
4. Apples
5. Peaches
6. Pears
7. Cherries
8. Grapes
9. Celery
10. Tomatoes
11. Sweet Bell Peppers
12. Potatoes

2017 Clean 15 List
1. Sweet Corn (some corn is GMO, so be careful)
2. Avocados
3. Pineapples
4. Cabbage
5. Onions
6. Sweet peas (frozen)
7. Papayas (Hawaiian papayas are likely GMO)
8. Asparagus
9. Mangos
10. Eggplant
11. Honeydew melon
12. Kiwi

13. Cantaloupe
14. Cauliflower
15. Grapefruit

Since you will be checking labels, be sure to look at the PLU number on the stickers commonly found on fruits and vegetables to distinguish between organic and non-organic. This is easy to remember as a 5-digit code with 9 as the prefix is used for organic produce and 4-digit codes are used for conventionally (non-organic) grown produce.

Interestingly, a 5-digit code with 8 as the prefix was suggested for GMO foods, but because it is voluntary, neither the produce growers nor the stores have adopted this code.

Grains

Grains are a significant source of calories in the standard American diet. Highly processed grains, such as cereal, bread, and baked goods, constitute the majority of our grain intake. Some advocate for a strict grain-free diet, which may be necessary for those with significantly dysfunctional digestive systems.

However, for most of us, a diet of organic, non-GMO whole grains is fine. I recommend avoiding gluten for the reasons listed below. For those with celiac disease, this also means avoiding oats. Other grains such as quinoa, brown rice, millet, and amaranth are generally well tolerated.

The most consumed grain is wheat, which permeates just about every aspect of our culinary lives. If you have ever "googled" wheat or gluten, you surely encountered a wealth of information about health problems caused by eating wheat, specifically the gluten found in this grain. In this section, I want to differentiate wheat and gluten fact from fiction.

A Short History of Modern Wheat

Humans have grown and eaten wheat as a major diet staple for thousands of years. It was a cornerstone of the agricultural revolution. It is important to note that while our ancestors consumed wheat, they did not seem to experience the health problems that we associate with wheat consumption today. Two early nutritional researchers, each focusing on local nutrition and its effects on health, did research among ethnic groups in different parts of the world.

Weston Price, a dentist, spent time among the peoples of the South Pacific and native tribes in Canada, both of whom relied on traditional diets. His observations of the students at a school called the Mohawk Institute located on the tribe's reservation is of particular interest. The children were fed a diet of raw dairy from grass-fed cows, vegetables, some meat, and bread made from wheat grown on the reservation. The children exhibited robust health, including their dental health, which was Price's primary focus. He tested this diet with lab rats. All those fed processed white flour developed diseases and suffered from obesity and tooth decay. The second group, fed whole wheat, were healthy, presenting none of the problems the other rats experienced.

Similarly, Sir Robert McCarrison, a British physician, spent time among ethnic groups in northern India and encountered the Hunza people whose diet consisted of grains (barley, corn, and wheat), vegetables, some fruit, dairy, and occasionally meat. He was amazed by the vitality and long lives of the Hunza people. Sadly, their health began to decline after the 1920s with the introduction of a Western diet of white flour, sugar, etc. So, there are examples of people doing quite well with wheat in their diets. The difference thus far is that successful wheat diets include whole grains, not white flour.

A Bad Choice with Good Intentions

In his book, *Wheat Belly*, Dr. William Davis attributes much of our modern health woes to the cultivation of dwarf wheat beginning in the 1960s. Wheat strains were hybridized to better tolerate pesticides and synthetic fertilizer, which increased harvests dramatically. This new wheat was celebrated as a solution to the world hunger problem, and to a large extent, it was very effective in this regard. Within a short period, most of the wheat grown in the U.S. and Canada consisted of this new dwarf form.

Several problems with this type of wheat have been revealed. First, it has very little nutritional value compared to its commercially produced predecessors. This compounded the pre-existing problem of nutrient loss due to the highly refined flours which become popular with the advent of steel rollers in the 1870s and chemical bleaching in 1950s. These two "advancements" left the flour devoid of much of the nutrients found in the wheat bran and germ. This turned a reasonably healthy, nutritious staple into an empty calorie-filler.

The second problem with dwarf wheat is that it is a "hard wheat," containing more gluten than many of the European strains. You may have heard of people who are sensitive to wheat in the US or Canada but eat wheat products in Europe and experience little or no reaction. The reason is that European wheat is of the soft variety, containing less gluten. Many European bakeries still use slow-rise yeast and prepare grains traditionally for baked goods.

Yet another problem with modern wheat is one associated with the pesticide, herbicide and fungicide chemicals used in conventional farming. According to data collected by the USDA Pesticide Data Program and compiled by the Pesticide Action Network (PAN), up to 16 different pesticide residues that have been found in wheat flour have been linked to cancer, hormone and thyroid dysregulation, birth defects, and neurotoxic effects.

Non-Celiac Gluten Sensitivity

Perhaps you have read news articles or online posts claiming that gluten sensitivity is a massive hoax or delusion. These authors, a fair number of whom lack any medical training, accuse people who don't have celiac disease but experience symptoms after eating gluten of being misguided. These authors have it all wrong. Research has established that Non-Celiac Gluten Sensitivity (NCGS), an adverse reaction to gluten without the presence of celiac disease, is a legitimate condition that affects real people.

Celiac disease is a hereditary autoimmune disease triggered by gluten exposure. Those with NCGS experience gluten sensitivity due to intestinal permeability, also known as "leaky gut." There is no autoimmune process with intestinal permeability. Instead, as a natural defense mechanism, the cells lining the inner surface of the small intestines create gaps between the cells to allow fluid to enter into the gut and wash away offending invaders. The cells, called enterocytes, are usually an impervious surface, much like a phalanx of ancient Roman soldiers with their shields tightly linked together, that prevents anything from penetrating the intestinal tissue.

Unfortunately, most of us have a weakened lining due to exposure to antibiotics, antacids, aspirin, and other medications. As a result, gliadin which is a part of gluten, can both cause and worsen intestinal permeability, allowing gluten particles to get deeper into the tissue. There the gluten is perceived by immune cells as something foreign that must be attacked. As gluten moves deeper into the intestinal tissue, it can find its way into the bloodstream, causing inflammation as it circulates.

Long-term gluten exposure with intestinal permeability will cause damage to the intestines. The damage may not be as severe as that seen with celiac disease, but it is enough to trigger many of the symptoms associated with NCGS, such as gas, bloating, brain fog, "food coma," cramping, and skin rashes. Anyone with thyroid issues should avoid gluten for this reason.

Ultimately, gluten is not a healthy food choice. Our ancestors had less exposure to it because the wheat they cultivated contained less gluten. Historical preparation methods limited gluten exposure even further.

Celiac Disease is Growing

Celiac disease is a genetic autoimmune disease triggered by severe reactions to gluten. It is estimated to affect 1% of the population; 97% of those with it are undiagnosed. Unfortunately, this disease is growing rapidly.

A ground-breaking study in 2009, commonly called the "Air Force Celiac Study," used blood samples taken from just over 9,000 young healthy adults in the late 1940s and early 1950s that the U.S. Air Force happened to have in frozen storage for nearly 60 years. These were compared with almost 13,000 samples collected in 2007-08 from those who were matched for gender and age. The goal of this study was to determine if celiac disease was becoming more common in the past 50+ years. The results were astonishing. Researchers found that the rates of celiac disease had quadrupled between the two sample groups.

A similar study looked at the rate of celiac disease among Finnish adults using samples from the late 1970s compared to samples taken in the early 2000s. Researchers found that the rate of celiac disease had doubled in that time. The search was on for what caused the rates of celiac disease to rise so dramatically.

Celiac disease is mistakenly associated with early childhood onset. There are plenty of cases of early onset, but Celiac disease can happen at any age if you are genetically predisposed. If you experience any type of digestive symptoms, I highly recommend getting tested for Celiac disease before going gluten-free. You cannot get accurate results with a standard blood test if you have been gluten-free for more than a month. If you are doing well eating gluten-free, you may consider completing a 23andme.com genetic test as it tests for the HLA-DQA2 gene, which is altered in 95% of those predisposed to Celiac disease. If you have an alteration of this gene, it is best to entirely avoid gluten.

Just as a reminder, gluten can be found in wheat, spelt, Kamut, farro, durum, bulgur, semolina, barley, rye, triticale, and oats. Those with non-celiac gluten sensitivity usually tolerate gluten-free oats. Those with celiac disease should avoid oats, however, due to the similarity between gluten and the protein, avenin, found in oats.

Meat, Poultry, Fish, and Eggs

The changes in vegetable, fruit, and grain production pale in comparison to those in meat, poultry, and egg production. Modern meat industry practices are inhumane and deliver unhealthy food to your supermarket. Fish is a healthier choice, but because of the pollution in our oceans and freshwater, pollutants and heavy metals taint our seafood. What should be excellent sources of protein have been rendered harmful to our bodies. Not all is lost, however, as we'll discuss the healthy options based on animals that are raised humanely and fed proper diets that make for high-quality protein sources.

There is much confusion about how healthy it is to eat animal proteins. This is entirely dependent on how the animal is raised and what it has been fed. Beef is an excellent example to illustrate this issue. Most cows raised in the U.S. are grain-fed for the duration of their lives. Grain is highly inflammatory to cows whose natural diet consists of grass. Eating grain causes massive weight gain for them with an increased fat build-up in their tissues.

Beef

Grain-fed beef has a high amount of arachidonic acid, a pro-inflammatory form of omega-6 fat associated with heart disease. Also, grain-fed beef is lower in vitamins. On the other hand, grass-fed beef is high in the heart-healthy omega-3 fat and has higher levels of antioxidants, including vitamin E. Furthermore, grass-fed beef has less fat overall. Much of the health objections associated with beef are based on grain-fed cows. When grass-fed, beef is actually healthy to eat. Most health food stores, including Whole Foods and several online services, sell grass-fed/finished beef.

Chicken and Eggs

We see the same issues associated with chicken and eggs, but the situation is even worse. Commercial poultry farming is extraordinarily unhealthy and inhumane. In the vast factory farm facilities that dominate egg and poultry production in the U.S., tens of millions of chickens are raises in stacked cages or are grouped together in small enclosures. Both egg-laying hens and chickens raised for meat are far more likely to suffer from diseases.

All of this can be avoided by buying pasture-raised, organic eggs and chickens. My favorite source is farmers' markets. Participating farmers almost always raise their animals healthily and sustainably. Many of the online services offering grass-fed beef also sell pasture-raised, organic chickens and eggs.

Seafood

Fish has long been a healthy source of protein. However, with the level of pollution in our oceans today, fish often contains high levels of heavy metals, medications, and other chemicals. It is commonly known that some fish such as tuna and swordfish contain high levels of mercury. This is typical of fish with longer life cycles.

Fish such as trout, salmon, sardines, and herring have far lower levels of mercury due to shorter life cycles. I recommend using a seafood-buying guide such as the Environmental Working Group's seafood guide, which includes a calculator to determine the safe amount of fish you can eat per week based on age, weight, and gender.

Pork

I've saved pork for last because I'm not a fan of pork and especially not a fan of pork raised in the U.S. As a whole, pork tends to have more toxins in the meat due to their nature as scavengers. They will eat just about anything, including other pigs. Pigs have fairly few sweat glands, which limits an essential route of toxin elimination. The digestive tract is another important route of ridding the body of toxins, which it expels through the feces. Pig digestion is rapid, and that's a problem. The short time in which a pig digests its food prevents the elimination of toxins effectively. Pigs digest food within 4 hours; compare that to the 24-hour digestive process of cows.

Modern farming practices only compound the problems inherent to pork as a food source. Pigs are raised inhumanely. Most are confined to cages that barely fit their bodies. In these conditions, they are far more likely to carry disease, which then can be passed on to the consumer.

The prevalence of antibiotics is a public health concern because antibiotic-resistant bacteria have become more common. According to a 2014 study conducted by University of Iowa researchers, households living within 2 miles of a conventional pig farm are three times more likely to contract MRSA (methicillin-resistant Staphylococcus aureus) infections than those who do not.

In general, I don't recommend eating pork because of the inherent health risks involved. This might seem like heresy to the paleo community and certainly to the Portland hipsters who seem to hold skinny jeans, ironic mustaches, and bacon in equally high esteem. But the conventional production quality issues of pork make it an especially bad choice. The only time you should consider pork is if you buy it from a local farmer who allows pigs to forage in fields.

Meat is inherently a healthy protein source, but because of modern farming practices and pollution, there are now health problems associated with eating meat. You must carefully select your animal proteins to ensure that you are not exacerbating the inflammation level in your body. Follow the guidelines outlined in this section to help you find quality meats.

Sugar, Frankenfoods, and Other Proinflammatory Foods

There are several broad categories of pro-inflammatory foods. What they all have in common, however, is that they trigger free radical damage in the cell and alter the production of proteins created by sections of genetic code. This leads to allergies, inflammation, decreased nutrient absorption, atherosclerosis, an increased risk of autoimmunity, and an environment conducive to tumor development.

Sugar

Our daily intake of sugar far exceeds what our bodies are capable of handling. In fact, since 1822, the first year that sugar intake was tracked in the U.S., our ancestors ate about 6.3 pounds of sugar per year compared to our current annual consumption of 105 pounds. in the United States.

Historically, our intake was lower because it was simply more challenging to acquire sugar. It was often seasonal (berries, beets, etc.), expensive, isolated (sugar cane), or there was a risk involved in obtaining the sweetener (honey). Now that these barriers have been removed, only impulse control stands between us and sugar.

Simply put, we overeat sugar. Reducing intake is critical for health improvement. The health risks associated with excess sugar are diabetes, obesity, and weight gain, but the harmful effects of sugar on the body are innumerable. I believe the right knowledge can change behavior, and I hope that this information strengthens your impulse control.

In Nancy Appleton's book, *Lick the Sugar Habit*, she scoured the medical research and made an extensive list of the health risks associated with our current intake of sugar. Here are few highlights from the list. Sugar upsets the mineral balance in the body by increasing intestinal inflammation and reducing absorption, which leads to deficiencies in copper, calcium, magnesium, chromium, selenium, and zinc. Sugar also increases the risk of cancer, including breast, prostate, rectum, colon, gallbladder cancers.

Most pertinent to those with thyroid conditions, sugar alters the immune system, increasing susceptibility to infections, and exacerbating autoimmune reaction by increasing inflammation.

To be specific, avoiding sugar means actively choosing not to consume the following sugar sources: sucrose (sugar), brown sugar, raw cane sugar, high fructose corn syrup (HFCS), corn syrup solids, dextrose, agave nectar (as bad as corn syrup), barley malt, beet sugar (commonly GMO), blackstrap molasses, brown rice syrup (high arsenic content), cane juice, caramel, carob syrup, coconut sugar, corn sweetener (GMO), crystalline fructose, date sugar, dextran, diastatic malt, diatase, ethyl maltol, fruit juice concentrates, galactose, glucose, inverted sugar (animal origin sugar), honey, malt syrup, maldextrin, maltose, maple syrup, molasses syrup, rice bran syrup, and sorghum.

Processed foods and drinks are the most significant sources of sugar intake, both in sugar content and consumption. I find that fruit juice and "supposedly healthy" energy drinks have a sugar content that rivals the soda pop that these drinks are intended to replace.

For example, an increasingly popular "natural energy" drink manufactured by Guayanki and found in natural health food stores, Yerba Mate Sparkling Classic Gold soda, contains 2 grams of sugar per ounce. Compare that to Coca-Cola's 3.16 grams of sugar per ounce. Yikes! This natural alternative has nearly as much sugar as the poster child of junk food. So much for a healthy alternative! This illustrates why it is so important to read labels. There are a lot of ways that manufacturers disguise sugar to make it look more wholesome and healthy.

Sweeteners are one of the cornerstones of processed foods and drinks. Historically sugar, along with salt, has been used as a food preservative. The food industry continues to use sugar as a preservative and in the process creates in its consumers a stubborn addiction. Let's take a closer look at the processed foods that feed this addiction.

Processed and Packaged Foods

It's no mystery why processed foods are so popular. They are convenient, and most of us are busier than ever. Not all these foods are necessarily bad. There are healthy choices due to the growing availability of organic, non-GMO packaged foods, but you must be sure to read labels, especially for sugar, salt, and unhealthy fats.

The foods that cause the most problems are those altered through chemical processing. They include foods containing high sugar and sodium, artificial colorings and sweeteners, flavor enhancers, preservatives, and other chemicals that are pro-inflammatory.

Typically, the production of these foods removes fiber, vitamins, minerals, and generally anything good for you. Overall consumption of these foods is at its highest level ever: 90% of our food budgets are spent on these foods. But there are hidden costs to all this "convenience." Science is pointing to heart disease, obesity, diabetes, etc.

Not only do these foods fail to provide nutrients, but some of the common ingredients found in them also deplete your body's nutrients. Two examples are the preservative disodium EDTA, which depletes minerals such as zinc and potassium in your body, and phosphoric acid, found in many sodas, which can cause osteoporosis and muscle cramps as it depletes calcium and magnesium.

Remember, sugar and sodium are key ingredients in processed foods as they help sustain the shelf life of these products. They may satisfy your taste buds, but at the same time, they trick the parts of your brain involved with hunger management, which often results in overeating.

Genetically Modified Foods, Pesticides, and The Thyroid

Genetically Modified Foods (GMOs)

The subject of genetically modified foods is hotly contested between the GMO supporters, who believe that GMO foods are perfectly safe and may hold the answer to feeding the world, and the GMO skeptics who question the wisdom and safety of splicing foreign genes into vegetables and fruits. I'm a member of the latter camp. Why is this relevant? According to a 2012 article written by the Environmental Working Group, Americans eat on average approximately 193 pounds of GMO food per person per year without realizing it.

The most significant concern is the lack of transparency concerning gene-splicing. We just don't know what type of new foreign proteins are to be found in these modified foods. There may be an increased risk of allergic reactions. Consider someone who is allergic to hazelnuts. If a gene from this nut were introduced into a fruit or vegetable, would this person be more susceptible to an allergic reaction? Some geneticists claim that since they can carefully select the genes inserted and that they have identified the genes and proteins that commonly trigger allergies, the risk is minimal. Unfortunately, there are no long-term studies on the effects of eating GMO foods on human health.

One principled concern that a few patients have raised is, "Do GMO vegetables that contain pork, and even human, gene splices undermine my vegetarianism/veganism?" That's a good question and one that's difficult to address on a case-by-case basis since every proposed GMO labeling law has been squashed by the GMO companies for fear that consumers would avoid their products. Ultimately, I would venture that GMO vegetables and fruit make vegetarianism impossible in the purest sense unless the gene splice source is identified. Personally, I think the cloak-and-dagger approach the companies have taken has been counterproductive, even for them.

Clearly, all is not well in the GMO world. First, there has been cross-pollination between GMO and non-GMO crops, and the GMO genes have won out, turning conventional crops into GMO crops. This begs the question: what will become of the non-GMO plants once GMO versions have established dominance.? There's no clear answer, but it is a concern for anyone who believes in the consumer's right to choose.

Directing our attention to the thyroid and the ability to produce energy, we find research that indicates that the pesticide Glyphosate, commonly known as Roundup, may pose a significant threat to your health. Crops have been modified to tolerate this herbicide, which is intended to kill weeds. The modification of these crops was meant to reduce the amount of Roundup used during the growing season, but we find that more of this chemical is being used and that many of its uses are "off-label," meaning that farmers are using Roundup in ways for which the chemical was never intended.

GMOs are still a big X-factor. They have yet to be proven safe since very few human studies have been conducted. Research using rats indicates that GMO genes may cause significant health problems. A French researcher, Gilles-Eric Séralini, published a paper in 2012 that found that lab rats fed GMO corn developed massive tumors in the liver, kidneys, and breast tissue. Therefore, if you are cautious about potential health risks, it is best to avoid GMOs. If you eat organic food as recommended, you are avoiding GMOs by default. You can learn more about which foods are GMO-free by checking out the "Non-GMO Shopping Guide" website.

Pesticides, Herbicides, and Fungicides

In the sections above, I briefly listed some of the problems associated with pesticide residues in non-organic produce. Now I'd like to go more in-depth to expand your understanding. I will use the term pesticide generically in reference to any of the pesticide, herbicide, or fungicide chemicals unless I specifically mention one of these chemical classes.

This topic is of profound relevance for anyone who has children or is looking to start a family because fertility and developmental issues have been linked to pesticide exposure. Most classes of pesticides are problematic, but I'll point out those that are especially harmful. Over time, they destroy our soil by killing off the microbes that produce valuable vitamins and minerals. Due to the widespread use of pesticide, we also see butterflies, bees and other helpful insects dying off en masse. As I mentioned above, be sure to use the Dirty Dozen/Clean 15 produce list to pick and choose among if you need to shop on a budget. If you have the means, I recommend buying organic produce to better protect the environment.

The herbicide Glyphosate has been used extensively worldwide since its introduction in the 1970s. In 1996, the first GMO crops tolerant to glyphosate were introduced. This resulted in a dramatic increase in the use this herbicide from about six million pounds to two hundred and forty pounds used annually in U.S. agriculture in just thirty years. Glyphosate was found to be especially damaging to the mitochondria, the source of energy production in the cell. Additionally, glyphosate appears to be linked to birth defects in Argentina, where the use of such chemicals is largely unregulated.

Studies have found correlations between pesticide use and thyroid disorders. Of particular concern is a class of pesticides called organochlorines, which includes DDT. These pesticides likely displace iodine, preventing the proper formation of thyroid hormones. One of the most disturbing developments in modern farming practices is the development of a class of pesticides used for soybean crops called neonicotinoids, which are linked to the mass devastation of bees. Neonicotinoids have been banned in Europe and in many countries around the world. Neonicotinoids cause disruptions of the hypothalamic-pituitary-thyroid (HPT) axis resulting in poor thyroid hormone regulation due to reduced sensitivity to thyroid levels in the blood.

As a whole, I recommend eating organic foods as much as possible. They are good for your health, your community (by supporting local farmers), and your environment (by supporting responsible agricultural practices). Furthermore, eating organic will help the detoxification pathways of your liver by reducing its workload. This will, in turn, support your thyroid function.

Is an Elimination Diet Right for You?

Many health experts recommend an elimination diet for those with Hashimoto's thyroiditis as a way of eliminating inflammatory, allergenic, and autoimmune-triggering foods from your diet. In many aspects, the dietary recommendations mentioned in this chapter incorporate elements of an elimination diet, but with a greater emphasis on making smarter food choices.

An elimination diet may be a good choice if you experience any form of autoimmune disease, chronic pain, inflammation, skin problem, or digestive problem. In these situations, looking for food reactivity is a smart first step.

There several different types of elimination diets, such as the Whole30, Vegan Cleanse, Autoimmune Paleo, and so on. They are all based on the elimination of certain foods for a set period of time, with special care given to the reintroduction of these foods.

The Basics of an Anti-Inflammatory/Elimination Diet

In an elimination diet, you restrict your intake to foods that are low allergenic and eliminate foods such as dairy products, gluten-containing foods, etc. The diet, in this restricted form, lasts for six weeks, followed by a careful reintroduction of possible allergens in small amounts to see if they trigger a reaction. Reactive foods are typically eliminated from your diet for three months.

The elimination diet is considered the "gold standard" for determining which foods are triggering reactivity, and thus inflammation, in your body. Food allergy/reactivity testing can be useful for finding specific foods that are problematic, but no test is 100% perfect. I'll discuss testing options below.

Among the most commonly recommended diets for those with Hashimoto's thyroiditis is the Autoimmune Paleo (AIP) diet. It is similar to the elimination diet described above. I'll explain the AIP diet in more detail below.

Other diets such as the Specific Carbohydrate Diet, GAPS, and FODMAPs diets are often adopted for the same purpose, but I consider them to be therapeutic diets for specific conditions. I don't recommend starting with these diets. Additionally, I don't recommend the ketogenic low carb diet for those with thyroid problems, as it tends to make thyroid symptoms worse. The ketogenic diet is most useful for those with seizure disorders. A modified low carb diet is helpful for people with diabetes.

Foods to Eat

Vegetables - Organic, non-GMO (nightshades excluded)

Fruits - All permitted (except oranges); eat a max of 2-3 servings per day to reduce sugar intake

Meats - (Beef, chicken, lamb, wild game, fish) - organic, free-range/grass-fed/wild caught, sustainably raised; avoid pork and shellfish

Grains - No gluten grains (spelt, Kamut, farro, durum, bulgur, semolina, barley, rye, and triticale), no corn; use organic, non-GMO, whole grains such as millet, brown rice, sorghum, amaranth, buckwheat, and quinoa; gluten-free oats - avoid if you have celiac disease

Nuts/Seeds - All are fine except coffee, chocolate

Beans/Legumes - All legumes permitted (except soy and peanuts)

Dairy Alternatives - Coconut, hemp, almond milk, etc. (*AIP only allows coconut*)

Fats: Avocado, avocado oil, coconut oil, olive oil, flax (better as ground seed since oil becomes rancid quickly)

Foods to Avoid

Vegetables - Nightshade vegetables (potatoes, tomatoes, eggplant, peppers, goji berries, bell peppers, and chilies)

Eggs - Eliminated as they are often reactive

Dairy - All forms of milk-based products (butter, cheese, cream, milk, etc.)

Grains - Gluten grains (spelt, Kamut, farro, durum, bulgur, semolina, barley, rye, and triticale), corn; (*note: the AIP eliminates all grains*)

Meats - Factory-farmed meats, pork, shellfish, no processed meats (salami, Bologna)

Sugar - Avoid all sugars (see sugar section above) and sugar substitutes

Nuts/Seeds - No coffee or chocolate *(note: the AIP diet eliminates all nuts and seeds)*

Beans/Legumes - No soy and peanuts

Dairy Alternatives - No soy or rice milk

Fats: Avoid canola and other seed oils (except listed above); no lard or butter

How to Test Reintroduced Foods Correctly

The reintroduction of foods is one of the most important aspects of the elimination diet. This is where the detective work comes in. After following the elimination diet for six weeks, introduce a single food for three days in a row, and look for symptoms.

Generally, there is no particular order of reintroduction unless there is a food that has been problematic in the past. Most people prefer to reintroduce their favorite foods first.

You should track foods reintroduced and symptoms experienced. New foods that trigger ANY symptom should be removed. Once symptoms have stopped, introduce the next food. Continue this process until all of the healthy foods are reintroduced. Eliminate any foods that are reactive for at least three months.

You may try reintroducing these reactive foods in the same manner described above after three months. There may be foods that are reactive for the rest of your life. In my case, cow's milk products and gluten remain reactive, so I just avoid them.

After completing the elimination diet, build your diet around tolerated foods in the healthiest forms you can find. Focus on eating foods closest to their natural forms: whole grains versus pasta or breads. The less processed the food, the better.

Use the basics listed at the beginning of this chapter as the foundation of a healthy diet. If you have Hashimoto's thyroiditis, it is wise to avoid glutinous grains during the reintroduction phase even if you are non-reactive.

Autoimmune Paleo Diet

I've mentioned the autoimmune paleo (AIP) diet several times thus far, and it's worth investigating further if you have any autoimmune conditions, especially Hashimoto's thyroiditis or Graves' disease. It is the most restrictive of all the elimination diets. In addition to the typical foods removed from an elimination diet, this diet also eliminates nuts, seeds, legumes, and grains. Like other elimination diets, there is a reintroduction phase to help you isolate which foods cause you problems.

AIP: Everything to Everybody

A point I like to share with patients feeling overwhelmed with the AIP diet is that this diet was designed for all types of autoimmune conditions. Certain foods commonly trigger specific autoimmune diseases. Examples include gluten and autoimmune thyroid, nightshades and rheumatoid arthritis, and milk products and type 1 diabetes.

There can be overlapping foods affecting more than one autoimmune condition, and for this reason, the AIP diet focuses on eliminating every possible trigger food.

Of the Autoimmune Paleo cookbooks, I prefer those by Sarah Ballantyne Ph.D., _The Paleo Approach,_ and _The Healing Kitchen_, but there are some good AIP cookbooks and many online resources for recipes. Another popular cookbook is Danielle Walker's _Against All Grain_.

Following an elimination diet, including the AIP diet, requires planning and strategy. Aspects to consider include new shopping habits, clearing out inflammatory foods, and planning meals for the week. Food preparation is a big part of the process. Many have found that a few well-spent hours on the weekend getting everything ready for the upcoming week makes the process much more manageable. Also, be sure to consult your family before starting this diet.

Chapter Highlights

- Organic vegetables and fruits are essential for improved health and should be consumed daily. Some individuals with autoimmune disorders react to nightshade vegetables.

- The petrochemical used in conventional agriculture have been linked to thyroid disorders and other diseases. Organic vegetables and fruit are recommended.

- Highly processed foods are pro-inflammatory, have little nutritional value, and are high in sodium and sugar. Reduction in these foods is associated with an overall improvement in health.

- Gluten, a protein found in wheat and other grains, is associated with digestive diseases and is a potential trigger for autoimmune thyroid disorders.

- An elimination diet can be helpful for removing potentially reactive and inflammatory foods from your diet allowing your digestive tract to heal. The Autoimmune Paleo Diet is a popular and effective diet for those with Hashimoto's thyroiditis.

CHAPTER 10

Best Supplements for Thyroid Disorders

Essential Nutrients for Optimal Thyroid Function

IN CHAPTER 9 WE FOCUSED ON IMPROVING YOUR DIET to maximize your nutrition. However, if you already have problems with your thyroid, chances are that you will need additional support using vitamins, minerals, and herbals to make you feel better.

In this chapter we'll look at supplements you may need on a daily basis and some highly effective strategies to help improve your energy and address other thyroid symptoms in a short amount of time.

I know this may be new territory for some readers. I highly recommend that you work with a qualified healthcare practitioner, especially if you are taking any medication. Be sure to check out chapter 12, where I provide recommendations on how to find someone who can help guide you through this process.

Please note: the vitamins, minerals, and other supplements discussed in this chapter are for informational purposes only. The information provided has not been evaluated by the Food and

Drug Administration but is based on research indicating potential benefits of the supplements presented. Again, I highly recommend working with a qualified healthcare practitioner before using any of these supplements.

The supplements listed in this section are those that I most commonly prescribe my patients. It does not represent an exhaustive list of all possible nutrients that might be used in a clinical setting.

Nutritional Deficiencies

Nutrient status and support is critical. A wide array of vitamins and minerals help thyroid hormones function correctly in the cell, and a deficiency in any of them will reduce thyroid hormone efficiency significantly. Some of these nutrients are needed to produce thyroid hormone itself, others help with the conversion from the inactive to the active forms of the thyroid hormones, while still others help transport the thyroid hormone into the cell.

Finally, many are critical ingredients of the cellular end-products that create energy in the body, which is one of the primary functions of thyroid hormone. Every step in this process requires adequate thyroid hormone and the vitamins and minerals needed to ensure that the body has the energy to function normally.

Many practitioners don't consider that when their patients take thyroid hormone replacement – T4 and/or T3 medications – it will increase the need for nutrients essential to the cellular end-products of metabolism because, with the medication, chemical processes are accelerated.

Most assume that a healthy diet ensures that all these nutrients are being absorbed and available to make this happen. This is a false assumption, and it is my experience that those who initially see an improvement in symptoms on thyroid medication, but then crash after a month or two aren't getting the nutrients needed to make the chemical products that, in turn, produce energy in the cell.

How to Identify Nutrient Needs

Throughout this chapter, I'll be discussing the nutrients that are most helpful for each of the different thyroid disorders and associated conditions discussed in this book. But before going any further, let's go over a few important points about using these nutrients. First, not everyone will need every nutrient listed in this section to improve their health. Second, many of the nutrients should be monitored via lab testing to ensure that you are absorbing the nutrients properly and that excess amounts are not inhibiting other nutrients.

Advanced Lab Testing

The best way of identifying nutrient deficiency is through comprehensive testing. Many deficiencies can be discovered through standard testing. However I find that using advanced testing, such as organic acids testing, is far more comprehensive and accurate.

I mentioned the organic acids lab test briefly in chapter 5 in relation to checking the efficiency of the detoxification pathways of the liver. The organic acids test, however, offers much more. One of the most useful aspects of this test is that it determines how well the cells' mitochondria are producing energy. This is a profound benefit as it can show us, albeit indirectly, how well the thyroid hormone is influencing energy production.

Additionally, this test can identify specific nutrient deficiencies, including cellular absorption of vitamins. Typical blood tests, such as blood levels of vitamin B12, indicate absorption of the vitamin from the intestines into the bloodstream, but they don't indicate if the B12 is entering into the cell. The organic acids test provides this information. Using an organic acids panel is extremely useful for optimizing your health. It has helped me un-cover additional nutritional needs that, when addressed, helped speed the recovery of my patients.

Two functional medicine labs are offering the organic acids panel, Genova Diagnostics, and Great Plains Laboratories. Both labs require that a licensed practitioner orders the test. Contact information about these labs are included in Appendix A: Testing Resources.

Making TSH & Supporting Pituitary Function

Before we can begin discussing thyroid hormone creation, we must first turn our attention to the production of thyroid-stimulating hormone (TSH) in the pituitary. TSH is a protein that requires a number of nutrients to ensure normal production and function. In this section, we'll review these nutrients. Conven-iently, many of these nutrients overlap with other aspects of thy-roid function.

Magnesium

Magnesium plays an essential role in the release of many of the hormones that the pituitary releases and TSH is no exception. A deficiency of magnesium will reduce TSH output, resulting in re-duced thyroid function.

Significant magnesium deficiency may have the appearance of partial pituitary failure. Several key regulatory hormones that the pituitary produces will be deficient. This primarily manifests as reduced adrenal and thyroid function. Magnesium is best monitored by testing the magnesium content within red blood cells.

There are two forms of magnesium that I prescribe to help improve magnesium stores in the body. Magnesium citrate helps relieve constipation and is usually taken at a dose of 400 to 600 mg daily. Be sure to start at a low dose to prevent diarrhea. Magnesium glycinate is best for those who don't need the laxative effect. An effective daily dose ranges between 400 and 800 mg.

Vitamin B12

Vitamin B12, also known as cobalamin, is essential for overall brain and nerve function. It also plays a role in normal pituitary function. Low vitamin B12, commonly found in those following a vegan diet, can reduce the production of TSH and also limit peripheral thyroid hormone conversion.

There are many different forms of vitamin B12. I prefer methylcobalamin as it is one of the most absorbable forms available. Supplements of lower quality will use cyanocobalamin, a synthetic form of vitamin B12 that contains a cyanide molecule. This is not dangerous to the body, but it does require the body to work harder to process.

I also recommend taking folate (vitamin B9) with cobalamin since supplementing B12 can mask the symptoms of folate deficiency.

Vitamin B12 dosage is dependent on your specific needs. Those with low thyroid disorders typically test lower for B12. Many have difficulty absorbing oral supplements. Therefore, I recommend sublingual B12 or B12 injections. A safe daily intake ranges from 500 to 1000 mcg.

Vitamin A

Retinol is the biologically active form of vitamin A and is essential for pituitary function. Vitamin A activates the gene that regulates TSH production within the cells of the pituitary.

Retinol is a fat-soluble vitamin, which means that an excessive intake can be toxic. It is not recommended to take more than 10,000 IU daily. I recommend monitoring retinol blood levels periodically when supplementing for longer than six weeks.

Zinc

Zinc is an essential mineral in the creation of thyroid releasing hormone (TRH) in the hypothalamus. Low zinc levels significantly reduce the amount of TRH created and released from the hypothalamus resulting in low thyroid hormone production.

Supplementing with zinc helps correct any imbalances. Supplementing with 25 mg of zinc picolinate or citrate daily is considered safe.

The Building Blocks of Thyroid Hormone

The following are vital nutrients in the creation of thyroid hormone within the thyroid. As mentioned in previous chapters, all of these vitamins and minerals are needed for efficient hormone production.

Tyrosine

Tyrosine is an amino acid that the body produces from the protein sources we eat. The thyroid protein, thyroglobulin, serves as the raw material for thyroid hormone and is made up of large chains of tyrosine molecules. Iodine atoms are attached to a small section of the thyroglobulin, which is then clipped off, creating thyroid hormone of which T4 is the predominant form.

Tyrosine deficiency is very rare and almost always related to a genetic disorder that is detected at birth. As such, I rarely see any benefit to supplementing with tyrosine.

Iodine

Iodine is a vital nutrient for thyroid hormone creation and is attached to thyroglobulin protein by the thyroid peroxidase enzyme (TPO). The deficiency of iodine intake has long been associated with hypothyroidism and swelling of the thyroid (goiter). Since the introduction of iodized table salt, we typically don't see massive goiters with iodine deficiency, though it does happen in parts of the world with low iodine content in the soil.

As mentioned in chapter 4, most cases of hypothyroidism are due to an autoimmune attack on the thyroid (Hashimoto's thyroiditis) and not iodine deficiency. Iodine has been implicated as potentially problematic for those with Hashimoto's thyroiditis because increased amounts of iodine cause the thyroid to produce more TPO enzyme. Since the immune system targets TPO in Hashimoto's, more TPO enzymes would trigger a worse autoimmune reaction.

However, based on my experience, I find supplementing iodine useful when found to be low. I will often test iodine to determine if it's low and recommend supplementation when appropriate. When Hashimoto's thyroiditis is present, you must balance iodine with selenium, which helps reduce antibodies and improve thyroid hormone conversion. For this reason, those with Hashimoto's thyroiditis would be wise to keep iodine intake under 300 micrograms (mcg) daily. Otherwise, a daily intake of 400 mcg is appropriate unless testing indicates a need for higher consumption.

Seaweed sources such as kelp, bladderwrack, and nori are high in iodine and have become popular as supplements and food sources. Of the three, kelp is the highest in iodine and nori is the lowest.

Some patients have expressed concern about the amount of iodine consumed by eating seaweed products, such as sushi or increasingly popular seaweed snacks. Both foods use nori seaweed, which is very low in iodine. The average 10-gram package of seaweed snack contains about 160 mcg of iodine. As such, nori is a good source of iodine at 16 micrograms per gram. Those with Hashimoto's thyroiditis or Graves' disease would do well to count nori seaweed consumption toward their total daily intake of 300 mcg.

Kelp contains approximately 8000 mcg per gram of iodine, far more than you need. There have been reports of thyroid swelling due to excess iodine intake from kelp consumption. Bladderwrack contains about 600 mcg per gram of iodine, which is also probably excessive if consumed as a food source.

Supplements containing kelp or bladderwrack should indicate how much iodine each capsule contains. Be sure to consult with a qualified health care practitioner when taking supplemental iodine.

Selenium

Selenium is another important mineral in the thyroid, second only to iodine. Measured by weight, it is highest in the thyroid. Selenium, as a key ingredient of glutathione, helps reduce free radical production that naturally occurs during thyroid hormone production. As mentioned above, it is especially crucial for those with Hashimoto's thyroiditis.

The best form of selenium to take is selenomethionine, which is safe to use at 200 mcg daily. It is best to test to determine your selenium needs.

Magnesium

Magnesium is an essential mineral that works in the thyroid to promote adequate T4 thyroid hormone production. As early as 1939, magnesium deficiency was associated with thyroid enlargement (goiter). Magnesium is also helpful for constipation and sleep quality. Consequently, I recommend taking magnesium at night for good sleep and a good bowel movement first thing in the morning.

Magnesium citrate helps relieve constipation and is usually taken at a dose of 400 to 600 mg daily. Magnesium glycinate is best for those who don't need the laxative effect. An effective daily dose ranges between 400 and 800 mg.

Important Autoimmune /Anti-Inflammatory Thyroid Supplements

In this section, I've included nutrients that are helpful to treat the autoimmune component of Hashimoto's thyroiditis as an antioxidant and to reduce inflammation because there is significant overlap. As we have discussed in preceding chapters, inflammation can be problematic at every stage of thyroid function. Thus, I will devote special consideration to anti-inflammatory nutrients.

Glutathione

As previously mentioned, glutathione (GSH) is a highly effective antioxidant agent found within your body's cells. GSH is especially important for the thyroid as it removes the free radical damage during thyroid hormone production.

Glutathione deficiency is common in states of chronic inflammation, especially in autoimmune thyroid conditions. Additionally, glutathione has immune-modulating effects.

In autoimmune disorders such as Hashimoto's thyroiditis, it helps to balance the immune system, reducing the autoimmune attack on thyroid tissue. Selenium is a key component in the formation of GSH. Selenium deficiency will eventually lead to glutathione deficiency.

The most significant challenge to addressing glutathione deficiency has been finding a supplemental form that is adequately absorbed. For many years practitioners used N-Acetyl Carnitine (NAC) and Vitamin C as means of increasing glutathione activity in the body, and it remains a useful treatment option.

Recently, however, new highly absorbable liposomal glutathione has been developed, which helps restore glutathione stores in the body. Studies have found GSH doses between 500 mg and 1000 mg to be most effective.

Selenium

The role of selenium is related to the formation of glutathione as indicated above. Studies have found that supplementing with selenium will increase glutathione production up to 40%. Additionally, research suggests that supplementing with selenium decreases the levels of TPO antibodies, reducing the destruction of the thyroid. The best form of selenium to take is selenomethionine, which is safe to use at 200 mcg daily. Selenium toxicity is rare. However, RBC testing is best to determine your selenium needs.

Superoxide Dismutase

Superoxide dismutase (SOD) is a potent antioxidant enzyme that works similarly to glutathione, reducing free-radical damage and inflammation within cells. SOD has also been found to help chronic joint pain. Like glutathione, SOD requires a mineral for proper formation, in this case, zinc.

SOD can be challenging to absorb. Stomach acid may destroy the delicate enzyme, resulting in little benefit. New forms of plant-derived SOD provide a stronger version of the supplement with significantly improved absorption. A word of caution: some of the lesser quality brands use wheat as the plant source, so be sure to look for gluten-free forms.

SOD potency is measured in McCord/Fridovich units named after the scientists who were involved in early SOD research, but most supplements simply list SOD in "units." Research has found that 5,000 to 15,000 units daily are effective in reducing free-radical damage. It is best to take SOD under the care of a qualified healthcare practitioner.

Turmeric

Curcuma longa, commonly known as turmeric, is an herb that has been used as a spice in India for thousands of years. Research has discovered that curcumin, a molecule found in turmeric, has various beneficial properties, such as antioxidant, anti-inflammatory, antimicrobial, and immune-modulating effects like glutathione discussed above.

As an anti-inflammatory agent, curcumin is very effective in treating a majority of chronic health disorders commonly seen today. I have used it clinically to help address everything from inflammatory bowel disease to Hashimoto's thyroiditis. Turmeric is one of my go-to supplements for reducing inflammation and free-radical damage. When combined with glutathione, turmeric can help reduce thyroid antibodies significantly.

The quality of a turmeric supplement is defined by its absorptive ability, which is enhanced by peppercorn extract, piperine, or a fat source. By itself, turmeric has more of an effect on the digestive tract and absorbs into other tissues poorly. Adding piperine extract to a turmeric supplement increases absorption significantly. For those who are concerned, peppercorn, from which piperine is extracted, is NOT a nightshade. Meriva is a patented turmeric extract containing soy-derived phosphatidylcholine, which increases absorption into the body.

Research has indicated that effective dosages of turmeric range between 1000 mg to 2000 mg daily. Turmeric has been shown to be safe at higher dosages, but there are reports of digestive discomfort at about 4000 mg daily.

Vitamin D

Vitamin D has been mistakenly called a vitamin. Technically, it's a steroid because your body produces it when the skin is exposed to sunlight. It is commonly low in those who do not get sufficient sun exposure. Supplementation is often the best way of increasing your levels.

Research has found that those with serum Vitamin D levels below 30 ng/mL experience more severe autoimmune symptoms associated with Hashimoto's thyroiditis and Grave's disease. Vitamin D appears to improve the sensitivity of the immune system, sharpening its recognition of the tissues of the body so that they are not mistaken as foreign. I recommend vitamin D3 supplements that contain vitamin K2 because vitamin D will increase the absorption of calcium and vitamin K2 directs calcium into the bones.

As mentioned previously, monitoring your vitamin D blood levels during therapy is important. Therapeutic dosing between 2,000 and 5,000 International Units (IU) is common but should be adjusted based on your lab results. For this reason, I recommend working with a qualified health care practitioner to monitor your levels and adjust your dosage accordingly.

Fish Oil

The oil extracted from fish is high in omega-3 essential fatty acids, which are strongly anti-inflammatory, have a balancing effect on the immune system, and reduce inflammation.

Eicosapentaenoic acid (EPA) and docosahexaenoic acid (DHA) are the two important components in omega-3, each having unique and beneficial properties. EPA is highly anti-inflammatory while DHA improves brain function, helpful for those with brain fog.

Other sources of omega-3 in the form of alpha-linolenic acid (ALA) include walnuts, flax seeds, and chia seeds. ALA is converted into EPA and DHA. I recommend fish oil over the vegetarian sources because the body converts ALA to EPA with only about 17% efficiency.

It is essential to read labels when selecting a fish oil for several reasons. First, you want a fish oil that is high in EPA and DHA, at least, 1000 mg and 600 mg respectively. Many of the lesser quality fish oils will list a higher amount of total omega-3 but skimp on EPA/DHA. Second, be sure to choose a fish oil with micronized filtration, as this ensures that pollutants and heavy metals are removed.

For most, the ideal daily dosage of fish oil is 1,500 mg of EFA and 800 to 1,000 mg of DHA. Fish oil may have a mild blood-thinning effect, so if you are taking any blood-thinning medicines, such as aspirin, please consult with a qualified health care practitioner to help you find an appropriate dose.

Guggul Extract

Guggul is a resin extract from the *Commiphora mukul* tree common in India and is frequently used in Ayurvedic herbal medicine. Studies have found that guggul has anti-inflammatory properties, which may benefit autoimmune thyroid conditions. However, if you are taking estrogen-based oral birth control or hormone replacement, you should be cautious using this herb as therapeutic amounts have been found to increase side effects of these medications. Please consult with a qualified health care practitioner to help you find an appropriate dose.

Iris versicolor

Iris versicolor, better known as Blue Flag or Purple Iris, is a popular garden flower that has anti-inflammatory properties. It has been used historically for reducing goiters and is helpful for stimulating glandular waste through the lymph system. Please consult with a qualified health care practitioner to help you find an appropriate dose.

Improving Thyroid Hormone Conversion

In chapter 3, thyroid hormone conversion disorders were discussed in detail. Now we will look at nutrients that will enhance the conversion of thyroid hormone from T4 to T3. As a brief review, the deiodinase enzymes are responsible for converting the relatively inactive T4 to the biologically active T3 by removing an iodine atom. While conversion happens in many of the tissues of the body, the primary locations are the liver, kidney, and intestines.

Several factors can cause thyroid hormone conversion dysfunction. These include reduced deiodinase enzyme activity due to nutritional deficiencies, excessive cortisol and inflammation resulting in increased reverse T3, intestinal microbe imbalances, and reduced liver function, commonly associated with liver congestion.

Selenium

Selenium, found in significant quantities in the liver and kidneys, two sites where the majority of thyroid hormone conversion takes place, is involved in the formation of the deiodinase enzymes that convert T4 to T3. As mentioned above, selenomethionine is the preferred form of supplemented selenium with a typical dosage of 200 mcg daily.

Zinc and Copper

Zinc is an important mineral needed during the T4-to-T3 hormone conversion. It is commonly deficient in about one-third of my patients. Common symptoms of zinc deficiency include decreased smell and taste, weak immunity, and poor wound healing. Supplementing with 25 mg of zinc picolinate or citrate daily is considered safe.

It is important to note that prolonged zinc supplementation over 50 mg can lead to copper deficiency. Most supplements contain a zinc-to-copper ratio of about fifteen to one. Copper deficiency is rare, but when it occurs, it can negatively impact thyroid function.

Guggul

As introduced in the previous section, guggul has been found to help increase thyroid hormone conversion. Additionally, this herb has been found to be helpful in reducing cholesterol levels and balancing blood sugar. Remember, guggul, and estrogen-based medications can interact, so please consult with a qualified health care practitioner to help you find an appropriate dose.

Ashwagandha

Withania somnifera, commonly called Ashwagandha, is another herb from India that has been used for thousands of years to increase endurance and reduce fatigue. It is classified as an adaptogen herb, meaning that it helps the body adapt to stress. As such, it has been found to be very helpful in reducing excess cortisol levels, which, in turn, improves thyroid hormone conversion.

Take note: there are several aspects of ashwagandha that raise concerns. First, ashwagandha is a member of the nightshade family, which means if you are reactive to nightshades, you may be reactive to this herb. Furthermore, this herb should be avoided during pregnancy and breastfeeding, and it is not appropriate for children. The typical dosage is 500 mg of an extract standardized to 2.5-5% withanolides.

Liver Detoxification

In chapter 5, we looked at how liver congestion, defined as a reduced function of the liver's detoxification pathway, can impair the thyroid hormone conversion process. In this section, I will present some of the most effective supplements for improving the function of the detoxification pathways.

Glutathione (GSH)

The anti-inflammatory properties of glutathione extend to the liver, where most of the detoxification in the body takes place. Glutathione helps in every step of the detoxification pathway process. It supports convert toxic byproducts of metabolism into water-soluble waste, which is easily excreted in the urine. Research indicates depletion of the glutathione supply in the liver can be a cause of liver diseases, such as fatty liver disease.

Superoxide Dismutase (SOD)

SOD is used along with glutathione in the phase one detoxification pathway. In this phase, which processes millions of molecules every second, toxins are broken down using enzymes such as SOD and GSH. Deficiencies of SOD reduce the speed, and therefore, the efficiency by which toxins are eliminated via the liver. Dosages between 5,000 to 15,000 units daily are effective in supporting liver detoxification. As previously mentioned, it is best to take SOD under the care of a qualified healthcare practitioner.

Milk Thistle

A highly effective herb, milk thistle, known botanically as *Silybum marianum*, has a substantial protective effect on liver cells. Intravenous milk thistle extract is used in hospitals to reverse liver damage associated with accidental mushroom poisoning. It has antioxidant and anti-inflammatory effects that improve detox pathway functionality. Additionally, milk thistle helps prevent glutathione depletion in the liver during increased periods of inflammation. Finally, milk thistle promotes the repair of damaged liver cells. I find that as a supplement, the most effective extracts of milk thistle are those with Silybum or silymarin standardized from 70 to 80%.

Dandelion

Taraxacum officinale, commonly known as dandelion, is often thought of as a weed. Despite its humble reputation, the root and leaf have been used medicinally for centuries to treat liver and gallbladder disorders. Specifically, this herb helps the liver by promoting healthy bile production and stimulating the gallbladder to release the stored bile, functions often impaired with liver congestion. Dandelion leaf has a diuretic effect, which may be problematic for those with low blood pressure and should be avoided by anyone taking blood pressure medication. The root is more commonly used for this reason. It may be used as a tea and is often found in liver detoxification supplements.

As dandelion has been shown to reduce the effectiveness of antibiotics, it should be avoided when antibiotics are prescribed. Similarly, it may influence the rate at which the liver breaks down other medications. Finally, those allergic to ragweed may react to dandelion. Please consult with a qualified healthcare practitioner to help you find an appropriate dose.

Ashwagandha

Research has also found this herb to improve liver detoxification pathways. It does so by increasing the activity of antioxidants, specifically superoxide dismutase, in phase one of the detoxification pathway process. Remember the precautions mentioned above. The typical dosage is 500 mg of an extract standardized to 2.5-5% withanolides.

Thyroid Receptor-Activating Nutrients

We became familiar with thyroid hormone resistance in chapter 3. As you recall, several factors can interfere with thyroid receptors actively accepting T3 thyroid hormone. Nutrient deficiencies, especially vitamin A and zinc, reduce the functionality of the receptors.

Inflammation and abnormal cortisol levels can also reduce receptor activity. Above we've discussed the anti-inflammatory supplements, which have the same effect at the receptor level. So, we'll focus on the key nutrients that improve receptor activity. Adrenal supplements will be discussed in the next section.

Vitamin A

The cellular receptors for vitamin A (retinol) are found deep in the cell on the surface of the nucleus, much like the thyroid hor-

mone. Retinol joins with T3 thyroid hormone to trigger DNA rep-
lication required to make cellular proteins. A deficiency of vitamin A reduces the ability of T3 to stimulate the metabolic activity
within the cell. Therefore, what might appear to be a T3 deficiency at the cell level may, in fact, be a vitamin A deficiency. Remember not to exceed more than 10,000 IU daily intake without
guidance from a qualified healthcare practitioner.

Vitamin D

Vitamin D, specifically the biologically active 1,25-vitamin D, has
receptors in proximity to the vitamin A and thyroid hormone
receptor on the surface of the nucleus. Vitamin D3 influences the
activity of T3 and the thyroid receptor assisting the process of
stimulating metabolic function through DNA activation and protein encoding.

Like vitamin A above, a deficiency of vitamin D reduces the
activity of T3, resulting in reduced cellular activity and an accel-
eration of the aging process as cells stop manufacturing the materials the cell needs to maintain optimal function. Since the body is
capable of producing vitamin D, I recommend a baseline blood
test to determine the daily dose of a vitamin D supplement followed by retesting every 6-8 weeks.

Zinc

The thyroid hormone receptor requires the addition of zinc to its
structure to form the shape that allows the T3 to bind to it correctly. Zinc deficiency can reduce the total number of thyroid
receptors in cells, resulting in reduced metabolic activity. Supplementing with 25 mg of zinc picolinate or citrate daily is considered safe.

Fish Oil

The omega-3 fatty acids found in fish oil stimulate the gene activity associated with the formation of beta type receptors, resulting

in increased thyroid hormone receptors in the cells. For most, the ideal daily dosage of fish oil is 1,500 mg of EFA and 800 to 1,000 mg of DHA. Remember the precautions above if you are taking any blood-thinning medication.

Supplements for Adrenal Health

We discussed in chapter 5 how adrenal gland dysfunction could hinder proper thyroid function. Cortisol, produced by the adrenal glands in response to stress and inflammation, can alter thyroid hormone conversion and trigger thyroid hormone resistance when elevated for prolonged periods of time. Adrenal fatigue syndrome can result from long-standing stressors and inflammation, which further disrupts the normal function of the body.

There are several approaches to addressing adrenal fatigue syndrome and cortisol imbalances. The first is through the use of adaptogenic herbs, a class of herbs that reduces the physical, mental, and emotional effects of stress on the body. All adaptogens influence circulating cortisol, either raising or lowering the stress hormone according to your body's need.

While adaptogenic herbs can be of great benefit, I recommend testing your cortisol levels using the adrenal stress index test first mentioned in chapter 5 to get a baseline reading, as you may need other supporting herbal therapies.

Ashwagandha

Ashwagandha has long been used to treat adrenal fatigue syndrome (AFS). It not only helps reduce high cortisol level but also improves the low cortisol levels seen in more advanced AFS conditions. If you already experience high cortisol levels, this herb is less desirable. Again, remember this is a member of the nightshade family, so if you are reactive to nightshade, proceed with caution.

Rhodiola

Rhodiola rosea, also known as golden root, is native to Russia, where the bulk of the research into the medicinal properties of this plant has been conducted. Another remarkable adaptogenic herb, Rhodiola is especially useful for mood disorders, including depression and anxiety. Several studies found Rhodiola to be helpful for fatigue associated with shift work.

Additionally, research has found Rhodiola to be effective for cardiac symptoms due to increased stress. Evidence indicates that this herb may help reduce high blood pressure and normalize irregular heart rhythms (arrhythmias). Traditionally, it has been used for altitude sickness. Research confirms the herb's ability to improve heart and lung efficiency during periods of physical activity.

The therapeutic dosage of Rhodiola is between 200 and 800 mg once or twice per day. The herb is well tolerated with few side effects. One minor side effect noted is a temporary increase in blood sugar at very high doses, which is normalized within two weeks of discontinuing. To date, research has not found any interactions between medications and Rhodiola.

Holy Basil

Ocimum sanctum is the botanical name for holy basil, also known as tulsi in India. It is a member of the mint family. Holy basil shows remarkable abilities in reducing inflammation and helping the body adapt to stress by balancing circulating cortisol levels. Holy basil also helps with the production of glutathione and superoxide dismutase. Additionally, it has been found to be helpful in normalizing blood sugar, cholesterol, and blood pressure.

Overall, holy basil has a calming effect and helps to improve mental clarity. One interesting effect of this herb is that it helps to reduce irritation associated with noise. I make a point of drinking tulsi tea daily as it helps me face my busy clinic schedule feeling calm and clearheaded.

Holy basil is available as a tea, tincture or in capsules. The standard dosage for Holy basil tinctures ranges from ½ to one teaspoon, taken two to three times per day. Capsule dosages are commonly 300 to 500 mg, taken two to three times per day. There is very little research regarding interactions between holy basil and medications.

Licorice Root

Another adaptogenic herb, licorice root is also known by its botanical name, Glycyrrhiza glabra. As an adaptogen, it has remarkable properties. It is highly effective in increasing and sustaining circulating cortisol levels. Seemingly contradictory studies have found that licorice root can also increase urinary excretion of cortisol.

On the whole, research indicates that licorice root increases cortisol overall. For this reason, I don't recommend its use for those with elevated cortisol levels.

Licorice root is beneficial for raising low blood pressure. In fact, it is one of the best supplements to address postural hypotension, which is lightheadedness triggered by a drop in blood pressure when going from sitting to standing. Studies have found that 200 mg dose of licorice root extract taken twice a day increases the blood pressure in those with chronic hypotension (low blood pressure) within a matter of weeks.

Because of its blood pressure-raising effects, I don't recommend its use for those with hypertension or who are prone to high blood pressure.

As an oriental medicine practitioner trained in Chinese herbal medicine, I view licorice a bit differently. First, licorice is commonly used in many herbal formulations but has a secondary role in the formula. For this reason, I don't typically use licorice by itself, as I find that the herb works better in conjunction with other herbs. This is another supplement that I recommend using only with guidance from a qualified healthcare practitioner.

Adrenal Gland Extract

The use of adrenal gland tissue has been used therapeutically since the 1920s with success. Most adrenal gland extracts are bovine tissues sourced from organic, free-range cattle in New Zealand. Overall, the extract supports and increases adrenal function by providing key nutrients found within the adrenal gland along with minimal amounts of adrenal hormones, such as cortisol.

You'll notice some similarity between the therapeutic use of adrenal gland and thyroid tissues. However, adrenal gland extracts differ from natural desiccated thyroid medication in several ways. First, these extracts are recommended because of the nutrients found in the adrenal tissues as opposed to the cortisol content found in them. In fact, only a few of the manufacturers standardize the amount of cortisol in the extract. Second, the extract is not a prescription medication; it is an over-the-counter supplement.

I often recommend adrenal gland extract combined with key vitamins for those with mild to moderate adrenal fatigue syndrome. Another application of adrenal gland extract that has been quite clinically successful is in the treatment of seasonal allergies. Combining adrenal gland extract with antihistamine herbs such as quercetin have significantly reduced allergy symptoms.

Therapeutic dosage for adrenal gland extracts is approximately 250 mg, taken one to three times daily. This supplement is well tolerated, but some may experience anxiety and rapid heart rate. This is seen in those with high cortisol levels and among those with severe adrenal fatigue syndrome, both of which can be determined with adrenal testing.

Vitamin B5

Pantothenic acid is a key vitamin for turning foods such as carbohydrates and fats into energy. It also plays a vital role in sex hormone production and the production of hormones of the adrenal glands, including cortisol. Additionally, it helps in the production of cholesterol and red blood cells.

The adrenal glands store a significant amount of pantothenic acid within the tissue. The prolonged stress associated with adrenal fatigue syndrome can deplete these stores, requiring additional supplementation to correct.

B5 is a water-soluble vitamin, meaning that excess amounts are excreted in the urine. However, taking more than 10 mg daily may trigger diarrhea and other side effects. Typically, daily intake is about 5 mg for adults, which is perfectly safe.

Therapeutic doses for treating adrenal fatigue syndrome can be quite high, up to 1500 mg daily, so it is imperative to work with a qualified healthcare provider to guide this process.

Vitamin C

Humans are one of a handful of mammals that cannot make vitamin C (ascorbic acid) from glucose. As a result, we rely on our daily intake of vitamin C-rich foods to meet our needs. Vitamin C is used in many biochemical processes in the body. A significant store of vitamin C is found in the adrenal glands.

As it relates to stress, vitamin C is depleted at a higher rate when cortisol level production increases. Interestingly, mammals that can produce their own vitamin C, such as goats, can make up to 100,000 mg of vitamin C per day when under stress.

The current RDA recommendations for adults is 90 mg. A majority of nutritionally focused healthcare practitioners find this amount to be profoundly low.

Most people well tolerate vitamin C, but high doses can trigger loose stool in some. Research has found 1,000 to 3,000 mg of vitamin C in divided doses daily is recommended for general health. 2,000 to 6,000 mg in divided daily doses is recommended for adrenal replenishment.

Chapter Highlights

- Nutritional supplements are often needed to replenish vitamin and mineral deficiencies, which helps improve thyroid function.

- Many of the same vital nutrients are used throughout the thyroid hormone process.

- Because of the complexity of finding the correct dose and avoiding any interactions, I recommend working with a qualified healthcare provider who can guide you through the process.

- Testing for nutrient deficiencies and monitoring ongoing supplement therapy is often helpful to ensure proper dosage and effectiveness of the treatment protocol.

CHAPTER 11

Lifestyle Changes
that Matter

As we have explored the different aspects of identifying and healing thyroid dysfunction thus far in the book, we have examined the different forms of thyroid related disorders, their possible causes, and the best ways to test them.

Also, we have discussed the importance of a healthy diet, medication options, and the most important supplements to rebuild and rebalance the body.

In the next part of our journey, we will look at one's life as a whole. In this chapter, we will identify and address sources of stress, discuss exercises that will help with thyroid recovery, and consider ways to ensure restorative sleep.

Stress - The Destroyer of Health

Stress, as defined the by the Oxford dictionary, is "a state of mental or emotional strain or tension resulting from adverse or very demanding circumstances." Stress is a common term used in our modern world and for a good reason: a lot of people seem to have plenty of it. It is important to note that though stress is usually presented as negative, there is such a thing as good stress. The terms, "stress" and "response to stress" were first presented by Canadian scientist, Hans Selye Ph.D., in 1936 as a part of what he defined as "general adaptation syndrome." He recognized a positive type of stress, "eustress," and a negative type, "distress."

Exposure to stress increases the release of a set of hormones – cortisol, epinephrine, and norepinephrine – from the adrenal glands, which sit atop the kidneys. These stress hormones help regulate the stress response that prepares you for "fight-or-flight" activity. This is how our hunter-gatherer ancestors survive the lions, tigers, and bears of their time.

For our purpose, we're going to look closer at cortisol as it plays a vital role in thyroid health. Cortisol itself isn't as harmful as you may often read about in the popular press. It is what you do with elevated cortisol that matters.

The eustress type of stress is usually experienced as motivation and drive to accomplish a task or goal. Cortisol rises and is released when the goal is achieved. Many high-performing individuals use this type of stress to their advantage. With distress, however, cortisol is rarely released, and the ensuing buildup can damage health.

After cortisol triggers a fight-or-flight response, some form of action is needed to "burn off" the excess. Historically, our ancestors were far more active than most of us today. By necessity, they found the means to resolve their stress and reduce their cortisol.

I will hazard a guess that most of you reading this book are not currently fleeing predators or facing some other peril as our ancient ancestors once did. If they were to survive, they had to act swiftly to deal with the source of distress. If they got away, they burned through the high cortisol.

In our modern world, sources of stress are not usually as immediate and dangerous. For most, sources of stress are often a matter of worries, responsibilities, and obligations. In these cases, you cannot use the fight-or-flight response that the high cortisol naturally activates without undesirable consequences. As a result, the cortisol circulates through our body with no natural outlet and causes damage. Today proper stress management involves appropriate physical and mental activity to neutralize high levels of cortisol.

The adrenals, the endocrine gland that produces cortisol, receive hormone production signals from the pituitary based on the feedback from the hypothalamus gland. This forms what is called the hypothalamic-pituitary-adrenal (HPA) axis. In addition to managing the body's response to stress and trauma, the HPA axis also regulates digestive function, the immune system, mood, blood sugar, energy, and sexual function.

When stress becomes chronic, cortisol levels are elevated continuously to address the inflammation that occurs. The inflammation, along with the constant stimulation of the adrenal glands to produce cortisol, slows down the hypothalamus and pituitary. Because the hypothalamus and pituitary also regulate the thyroid, we see a snowball effect that leads to a suppression of thyroid function.

Your Stress Inventory and Ways to Manage Stress

The stress inventory is a tool that I've been using for years in my clinic. I adapted this from Dr. James L. Wilson's excellent book, *Adrenal Fatigue: The 21st Century Stress Syndrome.* The purpose of the inventory is to help you identify sources that cause and relieve stress in your life.

Our modern lifestyle is one of the most unhealthy and stressful in recorded history. Chronic, unrelenting stressors in our daily lives are destroying our health and can be a source of the majority of our health problems today.

Ultimately four sources of stress affect our body:

1) Emotional (demanding work schedule, the birth of a new baby, the death of a loved one, etc.)

2) Physical (trauma, injury),

3) Environmental (pollution, pesticides, carcinogens, etc.)

4) Hidden sources (infections, inflammation, food allergies, etc.)

The stress inventory is focused on the emotional sources of stress, which those focused on thyroid and adrenal health concerns often overlook.

How to Use this Form:

I recommend getting a piece of paper, folding it in half lengthwise, and creating two columns. Label the left side, "Good for Me," and the right side, "Bad for Me."

<u>Step 1</u>
In the "good" column list all the things that you feel contribute to your health and well-being. These can be physical or leisure activities, eating patterns, exercise, relationships, work, family, emotional patterns, attitudes, beliefs, dietary supplements, and anything else that makes you feel good and contributes to your sense of well-being.

NOTE: do not list things that "should" be good for you, or which you do not find pleasurable or beneficial.

In the "bad" column list everything that seems detrimental to your health and well-being. Again, these can be physical, emotional, or attitude-based; they may be work or family-related situations, relationships, eating and drinking patterns, or anything you are doing or involved with that you believe is not right for you.

If some aspects of a situation are good and some bad, separate them. For example, you have a job that you love, but the grueling hours and fast pace are exhausting. In this case, put your job in the "good" column and the excess hours and high pressure demands in the "bad" column.

Take your time completing this form and use extra sheets if necessary. Your list for each column should have, at least, 20 items. Most people will have much more. Look carefully to see what in your life is working and what is not.

Step 2

Review each column and then circle the five most significant entries in each. Rank each of those five from one to five with one being the most important and five being the least. Now go back to the top 5 in the "Bad" column and identify exactly what about these items is so hard on you. Look at them under a microscope until you have a clear picture of the main things in your life that are compromising your health.

Select the worse (#1 in the bad column) and determine how much it is detracting from your well-being. Commit to eliminating this item from your life. Devise a plan for accomplishing this and the date by which it will be done. Write down your resolution and put it somewhere private, but in a place where you will see it often. If it's too personal, use a symbol to represent it and place it somewhere so that you will see it several times a day. Once accomplished, do the same with #2 in the "bad" column, and so on.

From the "good" column review the five positive things you circled and see what you can do to bring more of each into your life. By eliminating the negative emotional stressors and enhancing the positive emotional experiences in your life, you regain personal power and come closer to living your healthiest lifestyle.

Vitamin S - Sleep!

Sleep is a fundamental part of good health. In fact, you can't live without it. Yet I find that about half of the patients in my practice don't get enough sleep in terms of quality or quantity. They aren't alone. Nearly 50% of Americans suffer from poor sleep, according to the Sleep Health Index survey conducted by the National Sleep Foundation in 2014.

Data analysis by Northcube, creator of the popular Sleep Cycle alarm clock app, found that of their nearly half million users around the world, Americans had the worst sleep quality! Interestingly, Swiss users had the best quality of sleep, even though they averaged only four more minutes of sleep per night than their groggy American counterparts. App users in Canada, Mexico, New Zealand and Japan were also reported as being poor sleepers. Let's look at sleep in greater detail.

The Role of Sleep

The average adult needs eight hours of sleep per night to maintain normal body function. During the sleep cycle, the body goes into a repair-and-replace mode, in which growth hormone is produced and sent to all the cells. This promotes cellular repair and the creation of new cells. Additionally, cells work to reduce inflammation by creating anti-oxidants.

The thyroid is very active during sleep. Furthermore, a considerable amount of thyroid hormone production occurs during sleep.

Studies have determined that insufficient sleep (defined as less than seven hours per night) over the long term can lead to memory loss, poor judgment, obesity, heart disease, stomach ulcers, constipation, and depression.

As if that were not enough, it also increases tumor growth rate, prematurely ages you, undermines your immune system and may increase your risk of developing autoimmune disease.

Sleep Apnea and Hypothyroidism

Sleep apnea is a health condition in which the sleeper stops breathing for a few seconds. The lack of oxygen during these pauses in the regular breathing pattern partially awakens the person intermittently during the night. Morning fatigue and headaches are the result. The severity of the sleep apnea is reflected in the severity of symptoms.

There are three forms of sleep apnea: obstructive, central, and mixed. In obstructive sleep apnea, the airway becomes blocked. Central sleep apnea differs as it involves the part of the brain that signals the body to breathe. Finally, the mixed form is a combination of obstructive and central sleep apneas.

There is a clear relationship between hypothyroidism and sleep apnea as 30% of those with sleep apnea also have been diagnosed with hypothyroidism.

Even more concerning is a study in which over 50% of participants were found to have high thyroid antibodies. It is important to note that not all of those with elevated thyroid antibodies had hypothyroidism. This implies that sleep apnea may be a cause of Hashimoto's thyroiditis!

As indicated in the preceding paragraphs, sleep is vital for our health, and the lack of it, either in quality or quantity, makes us susceptible to chronic disease. It is essential that anyone with sleep problems look closely at possible triggers, including sleep apnea.

If you have been told that you snore or stop breathing during the night, it would be wise to be tested for sleep apnea. If you have been diagnosed with sleep apnea, explore your treatment options – there are alternatives to the bulky CPAP mask.

Insomnia

A Surprising Symptom of Low Thyroid Function

Insomnia is defined as difficulty falling or staying asleep and can have a profound effect on your health. About 30% of American adults report experiencing insomnia to some degree in the past

12 months. 10-15% experience chronic insomnia. Many of these people turn to medication to help them sleep. Unfortunately, a recent review by the FDA has found many of the over-the-counter sleep medications to be ineffective.

There are many causes of insufficient sleep, including poor sleep habits, increased stress, depression, anxiety, restless leg syndrome, medication side effects, and adrenal fatigue.

It's easy to take sleep for granted, that is until you don't get enough. One night of sleeping only four to six hours can impact your ability to think clearly the next day, and when one night stretches into two or three, then weeks or months, you've got a serious problem on your hands.

- Chronic insomnia is defined as poor sleep patterns lasting more than one month and is further divided into three subtypes:

- Chronic early-awakening insomnia: waking after a few hours of sleep

- Chronic sleep-maintenance insomnia: people who have difficulty falling back to sleep after waking, often several times per night

- Chronic sleep-onset insomnia: difficulty falling asleep

There is typically one or more health disorders that are the underlying causes of chronic insomnia. Based on my clinical experience, the most common cause is advanced adrenal fatigue syndrome (AFS). As you recall, I discussed this in detail in chapter 5. Here is how it relates to insomnia: in advanced adrenal fatigue syndrome low cortisol levels are found throughout the day but tend to be higher at night. This accounts for a common symptom of AFS, often described as feeling "wired and tired" at night.

An adrenal saliva test can help you determine your cortisol levels at night. If it's high, then specific supplements can reduce your high nighttime cortisol levels to help you sleep better.

Many benefit from using magnesium citrate as it calms the mind and body. Studies have found 400 mg an hour before bed improves sleep quality significantly without the morning grogginess associated with other natural sleep aids such as melatonin or GABA.

Steps to Improve the Quality of Sleep

If you are experiencing sleep apnea or elevated nighttime cortisol, you'll need to address these issues first. There are many things you can do, however, to improve your quality of sleep overall. The following recommendations are divided into three categories: 1) Optimizing your bedroom for sleep, 2) Preparing for bed, 3) Enhancing sleep through lifestyle.

Optimizing Your Bedroom for Sleep

Sleep in complete darkness or near darkness—this helps the light-sensitive pineal gland produce adequate amounts of melatonin and serotonin. This may mean installing blackout curtains, covering L.E.D. alarm clocks, eliminating night lights, and avoiding turning on lights during nighttime visits to the restroom.

Set bedroom temperature between 60° and 68° degrees. Sleep is negatively affected if the temperature is above or below the suggested temperatures.

Limit electronics in the bedroom. The Electromagnetic Fields (EMFs) generated by electronics can also affect your sleep quality. Keep all necessary electronics at least 3 feet from your body. Again, remember to cover any clock face to block the LED light. Personally, I unplug every non-necessary electric device in the house before going to bed. You should also disconnect the household Wi-Fi before bed as the signal can disturb sleep.

Loud alarm clocks disrupt sleep patterns. Being woken by a jarring sound, while effective, can cause stress. Sunrise alarm clocks are becoming increasingly popular —instead of sound, a dawning light, much like a natural sunrise, wakes you at a set time. One of the better-rated sun alarms is the Hf3470/60 Wakeup Light made by Philips

Beds are for sleeping. Avoid watching TV and doing work in bed, which can make it harder to fall asleep. Separate bedrooms may be appropriate if you have problems sleeping due to a snoring or restless partner.

Preparing for Bed

Going to bed by 10 pm is ideal as the adrenal glands recharge themselves between 11 pm and 1 am. Also maintaining a regular sleep schedule even on weekends helps the body establish healthy circadian (sleep) rhythms.

Fluids & Bladder: Avoid any liquids, at least, two hours before bed and use the restroom before sleep. Obvious I know, but you'd be surprised how often people don't do this.

Evening snacks should consist of a high protein source—L-tryptophan promotes melatonin production. Adding a small piece of fruit with your evening snack improves the transport of L-tryptophan across the blood-brain barrier. Avoid snacks high in sugar and grains.

A hot bath or shower before bed temporarily raises the body temperature. The subsequent drop in temperature triggers the sleep mechanism in the body. Also, wearing socks to bed helps improve circulation to the feet at night.

Minimize stimulation before bed. So, no TV or work projects for, at least, one hour before bed. TV has been found to disrupt the pineal gland function. Relaxing music is a much better choice. For those who suffer from a racing mind at night, journaling has been found to help clear the mind.

Lifestyle Changes for Better Sleep

Avoid caffeine and alcohol and check any medication you are taking for side effects that may affect your sleep. You may need to make adjustments when you take certain medication. I have found that many health conditions can be resolved naturally, eliminating the need for sleep-disrupting medications.

Relaxation exercises before going to sleep can help activate the rest-and-digest part of the nervous system. There are several of these exercises. My favorite is the facial muscle relaxation exercise, in which you start by scrunching up your face a second or two and then focus on relaxing the muscles of your face starting with your forehead, then the muscles around the eyebrows and nose, and finally the muscles of the mouth and jaw. I recommend visualizing the muscles relaxing as you inhale and the tension lifting as you exhale. I usually repeat this exercise three to four times until I feel relaxed and fall asleep.

The Importance of Exercise

Exercise is an import part of a healthy lifestyle, but many of my hypothyroid patients are faced with a problem. How do you exercise when you are always exhausted, especially if exercise makes your fatigue worse?

Unfortunately, there isn't a consensus among thyroid experts as to what type of exercise is best for those with thyroid problems. I have spent years sifting through research and have found approaches to exercise that have helped my patients. This section is written to provide you with guidelines for healthy exercise when you have low thyroid function.

Does Exercise Improve or Worsen Your Symptoms?

Because energy production is inherently low with most thyroid disorders, it is important to focus on the level of fatigue after activity. Carefully reviewing your response to exercise is important because changes in endurance, especially improvements, are helpful indicators of the direction in which your lifestyle changes and treatment may be heading.

Your response to exercise is more significant than the practical point of determining which overly fatiguing activities to avoid. Low thyroid function increases the risk of over-exercising. Because the body has a threshold as to how much exercise is beneficial, an excess actually causes the body harm.

A good example of this is running a marathon. If you aren't familiar with the origin of this race, it comes from Ancient Greece. A Greek soldier ran 25 miles from Marathon to Athens to announce the defeat of the Persian army. Upon delivering the good news, the soldier fell over dead from exhaustion.

Perhaps it's an extreme example, but the point is clear: too much physical exertion is problematic. For those individuals with low thyroid function, this threshold is much easier to cross than it is for others.

Over-Exercise, Cortisol, and Thyroid Disorders

Over-exercising is of particular concern for anyone with low thyroid because it triggers increased cortisol. We reviewed the role of cortisol in thyroid function in chapter 5. Suffice to say; increased cortisol can reduce thyroid hormone conversion and increase thyroid hormone resistance.

Those with low cortisol production due to adrenal fatigue syndrome will likely experience a worsening of fatigue as the adrenals try to release cortisol but fail to mount an appropriate response to the increased inflammation associated with strenuous exercise.

Additionally, strenuous exercise increases the use of electrolyte minerals in the body, such as potassium, sodium, chloride, bicarbonate. These electrolytes are likely to be out of balance in those with low thyroid function, and exercise could worsen this imbalance.

This is especially pertinent to those who also experience adrenal fatigue syndrome because the adrenal glands play a role in recycling the electrolyte minerals in the kidneys. The more severe the adrenal dysfunction, the more likely that electrolytes are lost through the urine.

Finally, because nutrients are often low due to poor absorption in thyroid conditions, the recovery from exercise takes longer. In such cases, the musculoskeletal tissues do not have enough building blocks to repair the damage that occurs with strenuous exercise. The result is long-lasting soreness and muscle fatigue.

Symptoms of Over-Exercise

Because of the concern of over-exercise with low thyroid function, it's important to recognize the symptoms of over-exercise. The most immediate symptoms – fatigue, mood swings, poor sleep, and brain fog – are noticeable shortly after excessive exercise and may extend across the following days.

Long-term results of over-exercise include loss of muscle mass and increased fat accumulation. Given our ideas about exercise in general, this may seem contradictory, of course, but the stress of over-exertion triggers increased cortisol, which, in turn, triggers fat retention. Muscle loss occurs when the body, in times of extreme energy deficit, scavenges muscle cells as an energy source.

The Paradox of Exercise and Low Thyroid

Because T3 thyroid hormone regulates energy production within cells, those with low thyroid function should expect less energy available for use. As a result, the beneficial effects associated with intense workouts (weight loss, increased endurance, sense of well-being, and better sleep) are not typically experienced with thyroid disorders. Instead, most of those with thyroid conditions shoot past their exercise threshold into the pro-inflammatory state of over-exercise.

Keep in mind that exercise is beneficial for you. You must simply adapt your exercise to match your body's ability to manage the stress associated with the exercise. Finding an exercise program that works is based, in part, on how affected you are by your thyroid condition.

As a general rule, the less endurance you have, the more careful you need to be. Those who are feeling better after changing their medication may be at risk for over-exercise, especially if nutritional deficiencies haven't been addressed. The key is, *go slow.*

Rebuild Your Body First

If you have been inactive and are looking to start exercising, it is essential that you start slowly. You might find restorative yoga or Yin yoga especially helpful as have many of my patients. This is especially relevant for those who have experienced severe fatigue over an extended period of time.

Gentle exercises such as the flowing meditative movements of Tai Chi or Qigong also greatly benefit those with low thyroid function. These exercises were developed in ancient China and have been used as part of an anti-aging routine followed by many Chinese elders. Both practices adapt well for the low thyroid community. I will discuss Tai Chi and Qigong in more detail in the next section.

Those who have better endurance – that is, they can get through their workday with enough energy to exercise afterward – will benefit from low-impact aerobic exercise and strength training. Again, with any aerobic exercise, make sure that you start slowly and gauge your response the day after exercise. If you are exhausted, then you have over-exercised.

The key to strength-training exercise is to start with low repetitions and breaks between sets. Not knowing your exercise ability, I advise you to consult with a personal trainer who has experience working with low thyroid conditions.

Yoga is also a good choice, especially yoga forms that emphasize breath work. I recommend a class in which the instructor is familiar working with those who have chronic fatigue conditions.

I do not recommend hot yoga styles, such as Bikram Yoga. While the heat might feel good during the activity, it is devitalizing, and there is a higher chance of over-exercise. Additionally, those who experience adrenal fatigue syndrome along with low thyroid will likely experience prolonged fatigue as the heat often worsens electrolyte imbalances.

Mindfulness and Emotional Restoration

Mindfulness and stress reduction have become a highly researched topic in mind-body medicine. Studies have shown numerous benefits associated with the techniques discussed in this section. What's more, many of the benefits discovered can specifically address symptoms related to low thyroid function.

The stress management techniques used in mind-body medicine are collectively called mindfulness-based stress reduction (MBSR) and include meditation, yoga, and body awareness practices. MBSR was initially created by Dr. Jon Kabat-Zinn who has researched the benefits of these methods. His work has inspired others to teach these helpful MBSR techniques. The website www.palousemindfulness.com offers a free MBSR training course online.

Having a master's degree in oriental medicine, I have found Qigong and Tai Chi helpful for calming the mind and reducing the effects of stress. Therefore, I have added these to the MBSR list of recommended activities. Both of these meditative movement forms originate in Chinese martial arts. They are incredibly gentle, however, and help strengthen the body, reduce stress, and clear the mind.

Benefits of Meditation

Meditation is the process of directing your attention inward instead of toward the outside world. The focus is often on breathing and letting go of thoughts of daily worries, tasks, and deadlines. It is a simple technique that helps you develop a quiet mind and lasting calmness in the body. Studies have confirmed the benefits of meditation and have found it to be a useful tool for anxiety. Personally, I think of it as a workout for the mind.

There are many online programs, smartphone apps, and guided meditations available for use. One of the best smartphone apps for both iOS and Android is the award-winning Calm. It is a paid subscription, but I have arranged a free month-long trial for my readers (www.calm.com/calmhealthtrial). While there are many excellent guided meditations, I have found a few specific to thyroid conditions. I consider the best to be Demo DiMartile's Thyroid Meditation.

Qigong and Tai Chi

Qigong is an ancient meditative movement system developed in China about 5000 years ago. Literally meaning "energy work" or "breath work," qigong is a combination of the internal focus of meditation and movement forms that help calm and strengthen the body. There are many different styles of qigong. Medical qigong would be best suited to your needs as this branch has been developed to address chronic illness. In recent years, medical qigong has grown in the US. A good resource for finding qigong practitioners is the www.qigonginstitute.org.

Tai chi is a form of meditation movement developed in the 15th century, which combines elements of qigong and martial arts and is highly effective for calming and clearing the mind, increasing energy, and strengthening the body. Additionally, tai chi can be adapted to any limitations you may experience regarding endurance, weakness, or pain. Tai chi classes are often easier to find because of its popularity. Additionally, there many videos online including <u>Tai Chi for Beginners</u> by Dr. Paul Lam.

Whether you try qigong, tai chi, or another MBSR activity, based on my experience, I believe you will find it helpful. I wouldn't be surprised if it made a tremendous difference in your recovery. Be sure to check your local community center for classes.

Take Time for Yourself

In the age of ever-increasing demands, making time for one's self is becoming rare. Among the trends that I've noticed as a practitioner is an eroding work-life balance. Many busy professionals become locked into a 24/7 work mindset. Add parenting to work demands and free time is often reduced to zero.

In all of the chaos of modern life, it's important to create time for yourself in which you step away from daily demands. Changing your mindset, focusing on your own well-being is critical for your health. If this approach suits you, try making appointments with yourself for pleasurable activities. Using the mindfulness-based stress reduction activities discussed above can a good way to build in "self-time."

Chapter Highlights

- The effects of chronic stress can be damaging to the body. It is important to find ways to reduce stress. Many effective tools help manage emotional stress listed in this chapter.

- While excessive sleep is common in low thyroid conditions, some have trouble getting a full night's rest. Any sleep problems must be identified and addressed to improve thyroid function.

- Exercise is important for optimal health, but those with low thyroid function are prone to over-exercise which injuries the body and worsens their condition.

- Yoga, tai chi, and qigong are good ways to restore energy and prepare the body for more strenuous exercise

CHAPTER 12

Taking Charge
of Your Health

Be Your Own Advocate

IN SCHOOL, ONE OF MY FAVORITE classes was the naturopathic philosophy class in which we studied the guiding principles of holistic medicine. One of my favorites among these
principles is "Docere," which means "doctor as teacher" in Latin.
But it goes both ways.

Over the years, I've realized that some of my most valuable
learning has been from my patients. No one person can know it
all, and if you have insight into your health condition, you should
share your knowledge with your healthcare practitioner. That
said, some practitioners may be more receptive to your input
than others.

Being your own advocate means standing up for your rights as
a patient so that you have the best chance to heal. This can be especially challenging in thyroid-related conditions because the
"party line" of conventional medicine has not evolved since the
1970s. This may require that you find a practitioner who is "thyroid literate," who will know more than just how to prescribe T4

thyroid medication. If that's not an option, you may need to educate your practitioner.

Where to Start

When choosing your health care team, you should first search holistic, naturopathic, and functional medicine professional societies' membership websites. This will help weed out those who are poorly trained as most require completion of a certification program before being listed on their site.

When you find a good lead, find out if the practitioner offers complimentary consultations. Most practitioners do, allowing you to get a sense of their approach, if they can help you, and if you feel comfortable working with them.

In many ways, the holistic approach to thyroid medicine is only now getting the attention it deserves. Of course, this often means that there is a steep learning curve for practitioners new to the approach.

To make your job a little easier, I've created a reading list that you can give to your healthcare practitioner (see Appendix B: Reading List). Of course, the realities of a busy practice and any semblance of life-work balance may delay this process in even the most open-minded of health care providers.

Ask Your Provider for Comprehensive Lab Tests

I hope that in reading this book, you have come to understand how important it is to look more broadly in order to experience lasting health improvement. The days of making a diagnosis based solely on TSH should be over. It is very important that a diagnosis based on all available data be made. For this reason, I recommend asking your provider for the comprehensive thyroid labs, including thyroid antibodies if this hasn't been done already. Likewise, a full iron panel and vitamin D is recommended.

Getting Your Own Labs Done

If for whatever reason, your practitioner is unable or unwilling to order these labs, there are commercial labs that you can order from directly.

All of these companies will contract with local blood draw sites or mobile phlebotomy teams in your area. I have created a list of labs I use (see Testing Resources). Several of these labs allow you to order directly without the involvement of a doctor.

Making Lifestyle Changes

Learning and understanding are important but applying that new understanding, putting it into action, is essential for making positive changes to your health. With that in mind, I urge you to develop a strategy for a lifestyle change.

Of course, I don't pretend to know your personal circumstances, but most people can find ways to start making changes that improve health, be it improving diet, stress management, adding vitamins and supplements, or starting a yoga class. Any positive change is a step in the right direction.

Priorities

As a way of offering guidance from afar, I have created some priorities in key categories that help provide infrastructure to make lifestyle change more manageable. Try to apply a recommendation from at least one of the areas listed below per week.

Of course, let your level of health and ability be a guide in this process. The goal here is to get rid of as many "steps back" from your life as possible so you can move forward toward a better quality of life.

Mental/Emotional

For many, the high stress of modern life can be a source of mental/emotional suffering. As I discussed in Chapter 11, there are a number of useful tools at your disposal, many of which you can do at home.

Among my favorites are the stress inventory, which I perform a few times per year, and meditation. There are many good at-home meditation options, DVDs, phone apps, and online videos. Creating time in your day for yourself is essential because humans need it to thrive.

Diet Change

The dietary changes recommended in Chapter 9 are important for removing potential allergic food, clearing out inflammation, and improving your nutritional status by eating foods full of vitamins, minerals, and antioxidants. The question is, are you able to go "all in" with this diet? If you can, then you should start to see improvements quickly.

But if you must pick and choose for whatever reason, I would recommend starting by removing as much processed and junk foods as you can from your diet. Next, switch to organic fruits and vegetables, healthy meats, fish, and eggs. Third, eliminate gluten. I'm sure some would argue that this should be first, and perhaps so, but for many this a significant challenge because gluten is in just about everything. Also, if you have any digestive problems, I recommend getting a blood test for celiac disease before eliminating gluten because you cannot get an accurate result once you've been gluten-free for more than 6-8 weeks.

Exercise

As mentioned earlier, exercise can be a challenge for those with low thyroid function. However, it is important because the body uses exercise to process toxins, eliminate waste, and stimulate the metabolism. Your ability ultimately defines both the type and frequency of exercise. For those who are deeply affected by low thyroid function, I recommend restorative yoga, which is very nourishing for the body, before attempting any other forms of exercise.

Keep Learning!

You are on a journey of health recovery, and it is important that you keep educating yourself to better help along your process and perhaps that of others. Some of this learning will come by trial and error, finding what works for your body. Additionally, there is a growing number of excellent resources in print and online. Support groups can be helpful for both your education and emotional support.

Staying Objective/Develop a BS Detector!

As you continue educating yourself, you will likely come across a lot of information online, some of which may be contradictory or just plain wrong. For this reason, I recommend developing a "BS" detector. Of course, "BS" stands for "Believable Source." This is especially relevant regarding home remedies that can be danger-ous and "health experts" who are better at selling their supple-ments than broadening your understanding of your health condition.

Support Groups - Pros and Cons

Support groups can be helpful because in them you have a chance to meet people who understand the health issues that you are ex-periencing. This can be of enormous benefit for those who feel adrift in their illness.

Most support groups have moved online, which offers a larger group of people with whom to share and learn. There are a few good support groups centered around thyroid concerns listed be-low.

There are also potential "cons" you may experience in support groups: smaller groups that have a very negative outlook on their health condition and cases of "the blind leading the blind," in which you may receive inaccurate information. I've seen patients who tried some far-fetched home remedies, which set them back considerably. This should underscore the importance of working with a provider who can determine the legitimacy of medical advice.

Good Online Resources

I've included some of my favorite online resources for thyroid education and support. There are plenty of sites online, and I try to keep track of much of what is available.

Hashimoto's Thyroiditis

I like the information offered by Dr. Izabella Wentz, author of *The Root Cause*, on her site: www.thyroidpharmacist.com. As a pharmacist and someone who has Hashimoto's thyroiditis, she has a balanced perspective.

General Thyroid

www.stopthethyroidmadness.com is a very informative, patient-driven website. They have a massive yahoo group, which can a be a good source of information.

www.hypothyroidmom.com is another good online resource, offering valuable insights written and curated by Dana Trentini, a blogger who overcame her hypothyroidism.

Finding a Practitioner Who Can Help

Throughout this book, I've discussed the importance of finding and working with a health care provider who understands the intricacies of correcting thyroid conditions. If you are not happy with the healthcare that you are currently receiving, you have options. I've created a list of different holistically and functionally minded medical societies that you can use to search for a practitioner in your area.

Of course, if you would like to work with me, I am available for in-person appointments at my Portland, Oregon clinic and online consultations for those at a distance. Visit my website for more details: www.drsoszka.com.

Functional Medicine Societies

Institute for Functional Medicine

The Institute for Functional Medicine (IFM) is one of the largest organizations of functional medicine practitioners that provides training in all aspects of health conditions, including thyroid. I am a member of IFM.

Functional Medicine University

The Functional Medicine University (FMU) is an online training program for healthcare practitioners. Much like IFM above, members are trained in treating many health conditions from a functional medicine perspective. I am a member of FMU.

American Academy of Anti-Aging Medicine

The American Academy of Anti-Aging Medicine (A4M), much like the Institute for Functional Medicine, is an organization with a strong emphasis on hormone health and anti-aging.

Association for the Advancement of Restorative Medicine

A smaller organization based in Canada, the Association for the Advancement of Restorative Medicine (AARM), is another functional medicine society that focuses on thyroid and hormones. I am a member of AARM.

Naturopathic Physicians

Naturopathic physicians (N.D.) were the founders of functional medicine way back in 1906. Our holistic perspective on health has now rippled out to other healthcare traditions because of the fantastic results we get. I am lucky to count myself among the ranks of this profession. The <u>American Association of Naturopathic Physicians</u> (www.naturopathic.org) is the national organization, which offers a provider search on their website. I am a member of AANP.

The <u>Endocrinology Association of Naturopathic Physicians</u> (www.EndoANP.org) is an organization of naturopathic physicians specializing in the treatment of endocrine disorders, including thyroid conditions. I am a member of the EndoANP.

How to Interview a Practitioner

Once you have found one or more holistically-minded practitioners, how do you pick the right one? What questions should you ask them? I've put together a list of questions and preferable answers to help you decide if the practitioner is a fit for your health needs.

1) **Which thyroid lab tests do you order? Are you willing to order a Comprehensive Thyroid Panel, including TSH, T4, T3, Reverse T3, and thyroid antibodies?** *If the practitioner uses TSH exclusively and is resistant to ordering the comprehensive test, then you had best move on because they aren't keeping up with the thyroid research.*

2) **When dosing thyroid medication, do you consider my symptoms, not just my lab results?** *The answer should be yes. As I've explained in this book, labs aren't perfect and don't capture every aspect of thyroid function. Symptoms are very important, as are other forms of testing. Your practitioner should consider all of these factors.*

3) **Is Levothyroxine the only thyroid medication you prescribe?** *The answer should be no. A good practitioner should be versed in using natural desiccated thyroid hormone and T3 medications, which would allow them to customize a medication protocol for your needs.*

4) **How often will you order tests to check my thyroid levels?** *They should recommend checking your thyroid levels of TSH, Free T3, Free T4, and Reverse T3 every 6 to 8 weeks while finding an optimal thyroid medication dose. Afterward, they should be tested every 4 to 6 months.*

5) **Do you use diet and nutrition to treat the thyroid? Will I need to change my diet?** *You want a yes to both questions. Many foods cause or worsen inflammation and lack nutrients. So, depending on your current diet, changes may be needed.*

6) **Do you consider adrenal function with thyroid problems? How do you test adrenal function when needed?** *You want a yes to both questions. Adrenal function is an important consideration with low thyroid function since they are both part of the endocrine system. Adrenals should be considered when thyroid symptoms return after a short period on thyroid medication. Saliva testing is the best method for testing adrenal function.*

7) **Will you order an ultrasound to check my thyroid health?** *Yes, is the correct answer. A baseline ultrasound is a smart choice if thyroid antibodies are high, or conversely when hypothyroidism is present, but there are no thyroid antibodies.*

If the practitioner can successfully answer these questions, then they are a good fit for your health needs. Continue to educate yourself throughout this process. Ask your provider about any recommended reading or resources as this expands your knowledge while testing theirs.

Next Steps and Final Thoughts

I want to thank you for taking the time to read my book. I hope you found it helpful and informative. The information I have shared has been the culmination of over 18 years of clinical practice and endless hours of education and research. I am very passionate about thyroid health and helping people regain their lives and enjoy optimal health.

I have written about the many aspects and the different types of thyroid dysfunction, the best thyroid tests, treatment options, and much more. But the ultimate "takeaway" is that there is a solution to your thyroid problem, one that, when applied, will help you feel your very best. Chances are that you have not had positive experiences in your efforts to improve your thyroid health. I say that this changes today.

Take Action

As I have said before, please take immediate action and incorporate the recommendations in this book into your daily life. They have worked for many patients and are very likely to work for you. Any steps you can make to improve your health will pay dividends in the future.

If you don't have a health care practitioner that you are happy with, be sure to check out the practitioner resources listed above. It will take some work to find them, but there are some brilliant providers out there who will help you restore your health and make changes for the better.

Learn More

Want to learn more about improving your health and optimizing your thyroid? Visit my website:

www.TheThyroidFixBook.com/bonuses

to get the free videos that accompany this book. Join my newsletter to get the latest information on thyroid health and news about my future book releases. I am in the planning phase of my next two books on thyroid.

Work with Me

If you like my approach to diagnosing and treating thyroid conditions, I am accepting new patients. I have recently integrated online consultations into my practice, allowing me to help those at a distance.

For those in the Pacific Northwest of the U.S., my clinical practice is in Portland, Oregon. Visit www.drsoszka.com to learn more about working together to restore your health.

Please Don't Keep Me a Secret!

If you received value from my book, *The Thyroid Fix*, please leave a review here: www.grade.us/drshawnsoszka.

Testing Resources

BELOW YOU WILL FIND MANY OF THE TESTING SERVICES used by myself and other functional medicine practitioners. The first section is a list of standard lab services that offer a full range of basic blood tests, including comprehensive thyroid panels. The second section contains a list of specialty labs providing advanced functional medicine labs. For each entry I indicate if the consumer can order directly from the lab or if a practitioner must first order the tests.

Standard Blood Testing Services

The following labs offer a full range of blood tests. Several of these labs offer direct-to-consumer services allowing you to order your own blood tests. This is helpful if you are unable to get your primary care provider to order a comprehensive thyroid test for you.

Ulta Lab Tests

www.ultalabtests.com

A direct-to-consumer lab offering comprehensive lab services. Rates are quite reasonable. They offer special lab panels and allow you to build your own test panels.

Principal Laboratories

www.principallab.com
Available to practitioners only. Principal offers deep discounts on labs, including comprehensive thyroid labs. I use this lab exclusively for patients who pay out of pocket. Typical costs are usually less than 20% of most major labs.

Direct Labs

www.directlabs.com
A direct-to-consumer lab that offers comprehensive lab services. Each month Direct Labs provides special discounts on a specific lab test, which is already at a reduced cost. On average, Direct Labs fees are usually less than 20% of most major labs.

Specialty Labs

Much of the functional medicine testing is through specialty labs such as the ones listed below. The tests offered by these labs consist of a myriad of advanced diagnostics tools, including comprehensive stool testing, organic acids, vitamin and mineral analysis, and environmental toxins testing. A majority of these labs are only available through healthcare practitioners.

Biohealth Laboratories

www.biohealthlab.com
Biohealth Labs offers a wide array of specialty testing, including adrenal, sex hormone, and Small Intestine Bacterial Overgrowth (SIBO) breath testing. I often use them for adrenal and SIBO testing. Available to practitioners only.

Cyrex Laboratories

www.cyrexlabs.com
Cyrex labs has many unique lab panels ranging from the most comprehensive gluten reactivity panel available to comprehensive antibody testing. These labs are very helpful for

uncovering the root cause of autoimmunity. Available to practitioners only.

Diagnostic Solutions Laboratory

www.diagnosticsolutionslab.com
This lab offers the GI-MAP test, which is one of the most innovative stool tests that uses DNA testing to identify the cause of intestinal infections, including viruses, bacteria, parasites, and intestinal worms. This has quickly become one my preferred tests for assessing intestinal health. Available to practitioners only.

Doctor's Data

www.doctorsdata.com
Doctor's Data offers comprehensive functional lab tests including heavy metal urine testing, detoxification pathway testing, and stool tests. Available to practitioners only.

Genova Diagnostics

www.gdx.net
Genova offers many very helpful functional medicine test panels, including Organic Acids testing and the all-encompassing, NutriEval. Available to practitioners only.

Precision Analytics

www.dutchtest.com
Home to the DUTCH (Dried Urine Test for Comprehensive Hormones) test. The lab has a strict focus on adrenal and sex hormone testing. They offer one of the most comprehensive reports available. These tests are very helpful for developing a deep understanding of adrenal and sex hormone health.

The Great Plains Laboratory

www.greatplainslaboratory.com
Great Plains offers advanced diagnostic panels focused on highly specialized testing for a number of health conditions, including

mold toxicity, fibromyalgia, autism, and chronic fatigue syndrome. Great Plains Lab also offers organic acids panels.

Reading List

I'VE CREATED A BRIEF READING LIST that you and/or your healthcare practitioner can use to expand your knowledge of the functional medicine model of treating thyroid disorder and their accompanying conditions.

Hashimoto's Thyroiditis: Lifestyle Interventions for Finding and Treating the Root Cause by Izabella Wentz PharmD

Stop the Thyroid Madness: A Patient Revolution Against Decades of Inferior Treatment 2nd Edition by Janie A. Bowthorpe

Stop the Thyroid Madness II: How Thyroid Experts Are Challenging Ineffective Treatments and Improving the Lives of Patients by Janie A. Bowthorpe (editor)

Why Do I Still Have Thyroid Symptoms? when My Lab Tests Are Normal: a Revolutionary Breakthrough in Understanding Hashimoto's Disease and Hypothyroidism by Dr. Datis Kharrazian

Hashimoto's Triggers: Eliminate Your Thyroid Symptoms By Finding And Removing Your Specific Autoimmune Triggers by Dr. Eric M. Osansky

Recovering with T3: My Journey from Hypothyroidism to Good Health Using the T3 Thyroid Hormone by Paul Robinson

Bibliography

Agarwal, R., Chhillar, N., Kushwaha, S., Singh, N. K., & Tripathi, C. B. (2010). Role of vitamin B12, folate, and thyroid stimulating hormone in dementia: A hospital-based study in north Indian population. *Ann Indian Acad Neurol, 13*(4), 257-262. Retrieved from https://www.ncbi.nlm.nih.gov/pmc/articles/PMC3021928/

Aggarwal, B. B., Sundaram, C., Malani, N., & Ichikawa, H. (2007). Curcumin: the Indian solid gold. *Adv. Exp. Med. Biol., 595*, 1-75.

Alzahrani, A. S., Aldasouqi, S., Salam, S. A., & Sultan, A. (2005). Autoimmune Thyroid Disease with Fluctuating Thyroid Function. *PLOS Medicine, 2*(5), e89. Retrieved from http://journals.plos.org/plosmedicine/article?id=10.1371/journal.pmed.0020089

Appleton, N. (1988). *Lick the Sugar Habit: Sugar Addiction Upsets Your Whole Body Chemistry 2nd Edition.* New York: Avery.

Arthur, J. R., Nicol, F., & Beckett, G. J. (1993). Selenium deficiency, thyroid hormone metabolism, and thyroid hormone deiodinases. *Am. J. Clin. Nutr., 57*(2 Suppl), 236S-239S.

Asik, M., Gunes, F., Binnetoglu, E., Eroglu, M., Bozkurt, N., Sen, H., . . . Ukinc, K. (2014). Decrease in TSH levels after lactose restriction in Hashimoto's thyroiditis patients with lactose intolerance. *Endocrine, 46*(2), 279-284.

Azizi, G., Keller, J. M., Lewis, M., Piper, K., Puett, D., Rivenbark, K. M., & Malchoff, C. D. (2014). Association of Hashimoto's thyroiditis with thyroid cancer. *Endocr Relat Cancer, 21*(6), 845-852. Retrieved from https://www.ncbi.nlm.nih.gov/pmc/articles/PMC4187247/

Bale, R. (2014, Oct 23). *5 pesticides used in US are banned in other countries*. Retrieved from Reveal News: https://www.revealnews.org/article-legacy/5-pesticides-used-in-us-are-banned-in-other-countries/

Barnes, B., & Galton, L. (1976). *Hypothyroidism: The Unsuspected Illness*. New York: Harper & Row Publishers.

Bates, J. M., Spate, V. L., Morris, J. S., St Germain, D. L., & Galton, V. A. (2000). Effects of selenium deficiency on tissue selenium content, deiodinase activity, and thyroid hormone economy in the rat during development. *Endocrinology, 141*(7), 2490-2500.

Beckett, G. J., Beddows, S. E., Morrice, P. C., Nicol, F., & Arthur, J. R. (1987). Inhibition of hepatic deiodination of thyroxine is caused by selenium deficiency in rats. *Biochem J, 248*(2), 443-447. Retrieved from https://www.ncbi.nlm.nih.gov/pmc/articles/PMC1148561/

Berlin, T., Zandman-Goddard, G., Blank, M., Matthias, T., Pfeiffer, S., Weis, I., . . . Shoenfeld, Y. (2007). Autoantibodies in Nonautoimmune Individuals during Infections. *Annals of the New York Academy of Sciences, 1108*(1), 584-593. Retrieved from https://nyaspubs.onlinelibrary.wiley.com/doi/abs/10.1196/annals.1422.061

Biello, D. (2010, August 6). *Genetically Modified Crop on the Loose and Evolving in U.S. Midwest*. Retrieved from Scientific American: https://www.scientificamerican.com/article/genetically-modified-crop/

Bilgin, H., & Pirgon, A. (2014). Thyroid function in obese children with non-alcoholic fatty liver disease. *J Clin Res Pediatr Endocrinol, 6*(3), 152-157.

Bland, R., Sammons, R. L., Sheppard, M. C., & Williams, G. R. (1997). Thyroid hormone, vitamin D and retinoid receptor expression and signalling in primary cultures of rat osteoblastic and immortalised osteosarcoma cells. *J Endocrinol, 154*(1), 63-74. Retrieved from http://joe.endocrinology-journals.org/content/154/1/63

Blank, M., Barzilai, O., & Shoenfeld, Y. (2007). Molecular mimicry and auto-immunity. *Clinic Rev Allerg Immunol, 32*(1), 111-118. Retrieved from https://link.springer.com/article/10.1007/BF02686087

Boelen, A., Wiersinga, W. M., & Fliers, E. (2008). Fasting-induced changes in the hypothalamus-pituitary-thyroid axis. *Thyroid, 18*(2), 123-129.

Braverman, L. E., & Cooper, D. S. (2013). *Werner & Ingbar's The Thyroid: A fundamental and Clinical Text* (10th ed.). Philadelphia: Lippincott Williams & Wilkins.

Brenchley, J. M., & Douek, D. C. (2012). Microbial translocation across the GI tract. *Annu. Rev. Immunol., 30*, 149-173.

Brown, T. R. (2015, May 6). *100 Best-Selling, Most Prescribed Branded Drugs Through March*. Retrieved from Medscape.com: https://www.medscape.com/viewarticle/844317

Brownstein, D. (2014). *Overcoming Thyroid Disorders - 3rd ed.* West Bloomfield: Medical Alternatives Press.

Brtko, J., Macejova, D., Knopp, J., & Kvetnansky, R. (2004). Stress is associated with inhibition of type I iodothyronine 5'-deiodinase activity in rat liver. *Ann. N. Y. Acad. Sci., 1018*, 219-223.

Burek, C. L., & Talor, M. V. (2009). Environmental Triggers of Autoimmune Thyroiditis. *J Autoimmun, 33*(3-4), 183-189. Retrieved from https://www.ncbi.nlm.nih.gov/pmc/articles/PMC2790188/

Caminero, A., Galipeau, H. J., McCarville, J. L., Johnston, C. W., Bernier, S. P., Russell, A. K., . . . Verdu, E. F. (2016). Duodenal Bacteria From Patients With Celiac Disease and Healthy Subjects Distinctly Affect Gluten Breakdown} and Immunogenicity. *Gastroenterology, 151*(4), 670-683. Retrieved from http://www.gastrojournal.org/article/S0016-5085(16)34713-8/abstract

Castagna, M. G., Dentice, M., Cantara, S., Ambrosio, R., Maino, F., Porcelli, T., . . . Salvatore, D. (2017). DIO2 Thr92Ala Reduces Deiodinase-2 Activity and Serum-T3 Levels in Thyroid-Deficient Patients. *J. Clin. Endocrinol. Metab., 102*(5), 1623-1630.

Cellini, M., Santaguida, M. G., Gatto, I., Virili, C., Del Duca, S. C., Brusca, N., . . . Centanni, M. (2014). Systematic appraisal of lactose intolerance as cause of increased need for oral thyroxine. *J. Clin. Endocrinol. Metab., 99*(8), E1454-1458.

Chen, J., Dai, W. T., He, Z. M., Gao, L., Huang, X., Gong, J. M., . . . Chen, W. D. (2013). Fabrication and Evaluation of Curcumin-loaded Nanoparticles Based on Solid Lipid as a New Type of Colloidal Drug Delivery System. *Indian J Pharm Sci, 75*(2), 178-184. Retrieved from https://www.ncbi.nlm.nih.gov/pmc/articles/PMC3757856/

Childers, N. (1993). *An Apparent Relation of Nightshades (Solanaceae) to Arthritis.* Retrieved from No Arthritis: http://noarthritis.com/research.htm

Chistiakov, D. A. (2005). Immunogenetics of Hashimoto's thyroiditis. *J Autoimmune Dis, 2*(1), 1.

Choi, Y. M., Kim, T. Y., Kim, E. Y., Jang, E. K., Jeon, M. J., Kim, W. G., . . . Kim, W. B. (2017). Association between thyroid autoimmunity and Helicobacter pylori infection. *Korean J Intern Med, 32*(2), 309-313. Retrieved from https://www.ncbi.nlm.nih.gov/pmc/articles/PMC5339455/

Combs, G. F. (2015). Biomarkers of Selenium Status. *Nutrients, 7*(4), 2209-2236. Retrieved from https://www.ncbi.nlm.nih.gov/pmc/articles/PMC4425141/

Cordain, L., Eaton, S. B., Sebastian, A., Mann, N., Lindeberg, S., Watkins, B. A., . . . Brand-Miller, J. (2005). Origins and evolution of the Western diet: health implications for the 21st century. *Am. J. Clin. Nutr., 81*(2), 341-354.

Cuomo, J., Appendino, G., Dern, A. S., Schneider, E., McKinnon, T. P., Brown, M. J., . . . Dixon, B. M. (2011). Comparative absorption of a standardized curcuminoid mixture and its lecithin formulation. *J. Nat. Prod., 74*(4), 664-669.

de Luis, D. A., Varela, C., de La Calle, H., Canton, R., de Argila, C. M., San Roman, A. L., & Boixeda, D. (1998). Helicobacter pylori infection is markedly increased in patients with autoimmune atrophic thyroiditis. *J. Clin. Gastroenterol., 26*(4), 259-263.

de Souza, J. S., Kizys, M. M., da Conceicao, R. R., Glebocki, G., Romano, R. M., Ortiga-Carvalho, T. M., . . . Chiamolera, M. I. (2017). Perinatal exposure to glyphosate-based herbicide alters the thyrotrophic axis and causes thyroid hormone homeostasis imbalance in male rats. *Toxicology, 377*, 25-37.

DePalo, D., Kinlaw, W. B., Zhao, C., Engelberg-Kulka, H., & St Germain, D. L. (1994). Effect of selenium deficiency on type I 5'-deiodinase. *J. Biol. Chem., 269*(23), 16223-16228.

Drago, S., El Asmar, R., Di Pierro, M., Grazia Clemente, M., Tripathi, A., Sapone, A., . . . Fasano, A. (2006). Gliadin, zonulin and gut permeability: Effects on celiac and non-celiac intestinal mucosa and intestinal cell lines. *Scand. J. Gastroenterol., 41*(4), 408-419.

Drugs.com Staff Writer. (2018, February 14). *Cytomel - FDA prescribing information, side effects and uses.* Retrieved from www.drugs.com: https://www.drugs.com/pro/cytomel.html

Drutel, A., Archambeaud, F., & Caron, P. (2013). Selenium and the thyroid gland: more good news for clinicians. *Clin. Endocrinol. (Oxf), 78*(2), 155-164.

EcoWatch. (2015, January 23). *15 Health Problems Linked to Monsanto's Roundup - {EcoWatch}.* Retrieved from EcoWatch: https://www.ecowatch.com/15-health-problems-linked-to-monsantos-roundup-1882002128.html

Editor. (2005, October 19). *All the Health Risks of Processed Foods - In Just a Few Quick, Convenient Bites.* Retrieved from SixWise.com: http://www.sixwise.com/newsletters/05/10/19/all_the_health_risks_of_processed_foods_--_in_just_a_few_quick_convenient_bites.htm

Editor. (2005, June 19). *Professional Compounding Centers of America.* Retrieved from Professional Compounding Centers of America: http://www.pccarx.com/

Editor. (2011, November 10). *Compounding Pharmacy Directory.* Retrieved from Compounding Pharmacies: http://www.compoundingpharmacies.org/useful-resources/state-associations/

Editor. (2012, July 12). *International Academy of Compounding Pharmacists.* Retrieved from International Academy of Compounding Pharmacists: http://www.iacprx.org/

Editor. (2017, March 17). *How can I safely consume seaweed?* Retrieved from Examine.com: https://examine.com/nutrition/how-can-i-safely-consume-seaweed/

El Asmar, R., Panigrahi, P., Bamford, P., Berti, I., Not, T., Coppa, G. V., . . . El Asmar, R. (2002). Host-dependent zonulin secretion causes the impairment of the small intestine barrier function after bacterial exposure. *Gastroenterology, 123*(5), 1607-1615.

Elsegood, L. (2016). *The LDN Book: How a Little-Known Generic Drug — Low Dose Naltrexone — Could Revolutionize Treatment for Autoimmune Diseases, Cancer, Autism, Depression, and More.* White River Junction: Chelsea Green Publishing.

Enderlin, V., Alfos, S., Pallet, V., Garcin, H., Azais-Braesco, V., Jaffard, R., & Higueret, P. (1997). Aging decreases the abundance of retinoic acid (RAR) and triiodothyronine (TR) nuclear receptor mRNA in rat brain: effect of the administration of retinoids. *FEBS Lett., 412*(3), 629-632.

EWG. (2017, January 2). *EWG's 2017 Shopper's Guide to Pesticides in Produce.* Retrieved from Environmental Working Group: https://www.ewg.org/foodnews/

Fasano, A. (2012). Intestinal Permeability and Its Regulation by Zonulin: Diagnostic and Therapeutic Implications. *Clinical Gastroenterology and Hepatology, 10*(10), 1096-1100. Retrieved from http://www.cghjournal.org/article/S1542-3565(12)00932-9/fulltext

Fasano, A. e. (2015). Nonceliac Gluten Sensitivity. *Gastroenterology, 148*(6), 1195 - 1204. Retrieved from http://www.gastrojournal.org/article/S0016-5085(15)00029-3/abstract?referrer=http%3A%2F%2Fgut.bmj.com%2Fcontent%2Fearly%2F2016%2F07%2F21%2Fgutjnl-2016-311964.full

Fenwick, G. R., Heaney, R. K., & Mullin, W. J. (1983). Glucosinolates and their breakdown products in food and food plants. *Crit Rev Food Sci Nutr, 18*(2), 123-201.

Frahlich, E., & Wahl, R. (2017). Thyroid Autoimmunity: Role of Anti-thyroid Antibodies in Thyroid and Extra-Thyroidal Diseases. *Front Immunol, 8,* 521.

Freake, H. C., Govoni, K. E., Guda, K., Huang, C., & Zinn, S. A. (2001). Actions and interactions of thyroid hormone and zinc status in growing rats. *J. Nutr., 131*(4), 1135-1141.

Friedman ND, M. (2014). *Naturopathic Endocrinology.* Lady Lake: Muskeegee Medical Publishing Company.

Friedman, M. (2013, October). *Thyroid Autoimmune Disease.* Retrieved from Association for the Advancement of Restorative Medicine: https://restorativemedicine.org/journal/thyroid-autoimmune-disease/

Fukata, S., Brent, G. A., & Sugawara, M. (2005). Resistance to Thyroid Hormone in Hashimoto's Thyroiditis. *New England Journal of Medicine, 352*(5), 517-518. Retrieved from http://dx.doi.org/10.1056/NEJM200502033520523

Gardner, D. G., & Shoback, D. (2011). *Greenspan's Basic and Clinical Endocrinology, Ninth Edition* (9th ed.). New York: McGraw Hill/Lange.

Gartner, R., Gasnier, B. C., Dietrich, J. W., Krebs, B., & Angstwurm, M. W. (2002). Selenium Supplementation in Patients with Autoimmune Thyroiditis Decreases Thyroid Peroxidase Antibodies Concentrations. *J Clin Endocrinol Metab, 87*(4), 1687-1691. Retrieved from https://academic.oup.com/jcem/article/87/4/1687/2374966

Goldner, W. S., Sandler, D. P., Yu, F., Hoppin, J. A., Kamel, F., & LeVan, T. D. (2010). Pesticide Use and Thyroid Disease Among Women in the Agricultural Health Study. *Am J Epidemiol, 171*(4), 455-464. Retrieved from https://academic.oup.com/aje/article/171/4/455/157410

Grani, G., Carbotta, G., Nesca, A., D'Alessandri, M., Vitale, M., Del Sordo, M., & Fumarola, A. (2015). A comprehensive score to diagnose Hashimoto's thyroiditis: a proposal. *Endocrine, 49*(2), 361-365.

Gruner, T., & Arthur, R. (2012). The accuracy of the Zinc Taste Test method. *J Altern Complement Med, 18*(6), 541-550.

Guayaki. (2018, January 13). *Classic Gold Sparkling Mate [Case of 12]*. Retrieved from guayaki.com: http://guayaki.com/product/2516/Classic-Gold-Sparkling-Mate-%3Cbr%3E-%5BCase-of-12%5D.html

Gullo, D., Latina, A., Frasca, F., Le Moli, R., Pellegriti, G., & Vigneri, R. (2011, August 1). *Levothyroxine Monotherapy Cannot Guarantee Euthyroidism in All Athyreotic Patients*. Retrieved from Pubmed: https://www.ncbi.nlm.nih.gov/pmc/articles/PMC3148220/

Guo, T.-W., Zhang, F.-C., Yang, M.-S., Gao, X.-C., Bian, L., Duan, S.-W., . . . He, L. (2004). Positive association of the DIO2 (deiodinase type 2) gene with mental retardation in the iodine-deficient areas of China. *J Med Genet, 41*(8), 585-590.

Gupta, S. C., Patchva, S., & Aggarwal, B. B. (2012). Therapeutic Roles of Curcumin: Lessons Learned from Clinical Trials. *AAPS J, 15*(1), 195-218. Retrieved from https://www.ncbi.nlm.nih.gov/pmc/articles/PMC3535097/

Ha, H. R., Stieger, B., Grassi, G., Altorfer, H. R., & Follath, F. (2000). Structure-effect relationships of amiodarone analogues on the inhibition of thyroxine deiodination. *Eur. J. Clin. Pharmacol., 55*(11-12), 807-814.

Hafling, D. B., Chavantes, M. C., Juliano, A. G., Cerri, G. G., Knobel, M., Yoshimura, E. M., & Chammas, M. C. (2013). Low-level laser in the treatment of patients with hypothyroidism induced by chronic autoimmune thyroiditis: a randomized, placebo-controlled clinical trial. *Lasers Med Sci, 28*(3), 743-753.

Hanai, H., & Sugimoto, K. (2009). Curcumin has bright prospects for the treatment of inflammatory bowel disease. *Curr. Pharm. Des., 15*(18), 2087-2094.

Heaney, R. P. (2011). Assessing vitamin D status. *Current Opinion in Clinical Nutrition & Metabolic Care, 14*(5), 440. Retrieved from https://journals.lww.com/co-clinicalnutrition/Abstract/2011/09000/Assessing_vitamin_D_status.6.aspx

Heyman, A., Yang, J., & Bowthorpe, J. A. (2014). *Stop the Thyroid Madness II: How Thyroid Experts Are Challenging Ineffective Treatments and Improving the Lives of Patients.* Dolores: Laughing Grape Publishing.

Hidal, J. T., & Kaplan, M. M. (1988). Inhibition of thyroxine 5'-deiodination type II in cultured human placental cells by cortisol, insulin, 3', 5'-cyclic adenosine monophosphate, and butyrate. *Metab. Clin. Exp., 37*(7), 664-668.

Hou, Y., Sun, W., Zhang, C., Wang, T., Guo, X., Wu, L., . . . Liu, T. (2017). Meta-analysis of the correlation between Helicobacter pylori infection and autoimmune thyroid diseases. *Oncotarget, 8*(70), 115691-115700.

Howe, C. M., Berrill, M., Pauli, B. D., Helbing, C. C., Werry, K., & Veldhoen, N. (2004). Toxicity of glyphosate-based pesticides to four North American frog species. *Environ. Toxicol. Chem., 23*(8), 1928-1938.

Huang, S. A. (2005). Physiology and pathophysiology of type 3 deiodinase in humans. *Thyroid, 15*(8), 875-881.

Huang, S., Dorfman, D., Genest, D., Salvatore, D., & Larsen, P. (2003). Type 3 iodothyronine deiodinase is highly expressed in the human uteroplacental unit and in fetal epithelium. *J. Clin. Endocrinol. Metab., 88*(3), 1384-1388.

Huang, X., Liu, X., & Yu, Y. (2017). Depression and Chronic Liver Diseases: Are There Shared Underlying Mechanisms? *Front*

Mol Neurosci, 10, 10, 134. Retrieved from
https://www.ncbi.nlm.nih.gov/pmc/articles/PMC5420567/

Iddah, M. A., & Macharia, B. N. (2013). Autoimmune Thyroid
Disorders. *Endocrinology, 2013*. Retrieved from
https://www.ncbi.nlm.nih.gov/pmc/articles/PMC3710642/

Immune Health Sciences. (2015, April 14). *Superoxide dismutase
(SOD)*. Retrieved from Immune Health Sciences:
http://www.immunehealthscience.com/superoxide-
dismutase.html

Jager, R., Lowery, R. P., Calvanese, A. V., Joy, J. M., Purpura, M., &
Wilson, J. M. (2014). Comparative absorption of curcumin
formulations. *Nutr J, 13*, 11. Retrieved from
https://www.ncbi.nlm.nih.gov/pmc/articles/PMC3918227/

Jones, J. E., Desper, P. C., Shane, S. R., & Flink, E. B. (1966).
Magnesium metabolism in hyperthyroidism and
hypothyroidism. *J Clin Invest, 45*(6), 891-900. Retrieved
from
https://www.ncbi.nlm.nih.gov/pmc/articles/PMC292768/

Kam, M., & Lam, D. (2012). *Adrenal Fatigue Syndrome - Reclaim Your
Energy and Vitality with Clinically Proven Natural Programs*.
Loma Linda: Adrenal Institue Press.

Kavvoura, F. K., Akamizu, T., Awata, T., Ban, Y., Chistiakov, D. A.,
Frydecka, I., . . . Ioannidis, J. P. (2007). Cytotoxic T-
lymphocyte associated antigen 4 gene polymorphisms and
autoimmune thyroid disease: a meta-analysis. *J. Clin.
Endocrinol. Metab., 92*(8), 3162-3170.

Khaliq, W., Andreis, D., Kleyman, A., Graler, M., & Singer, M.
(2015). Reductions in tyrosine levels are associated with
thyroid hormone and catecholamine disturbances in sepsis.
Intensive Care Med Exp, 3(Suppl 1), A686. Retrieved from
https://www.ncbi.nlm.nih.gov/pmc/articles/PMC4798095/

Kharrazian, D. (2010). *Why Do I Still Have Thyroid Symptoms? when My Lab Tests Are Normal: a Revolutionary Breakthrough in Understanding Hashimoto's Disease and Hypothyroidism.* Garden City: Morgan James Publishing, LLC.

Khatiwada, S., Gelal, B., Baral, N., & Lamsal, M. (2016). Association between iron status and thyroid function in {Nepalese} children. *Thyroid Res, 9,* 9, 2. Retrieved from https://www.ncbi.nlm.nih.gov/pmc/articles/PMC4729155/

Kiefer, D. (2006, June). *Superoxide Dismutase: Boosting the Body's Primary Antioxidant Defense.* Retrieved from Life Extension: http://www.lifeextension.com/magazine/2006/6/report_s od/Page-01

Kim, E., Lim, D., Baek, K., Lee, J., Kim, M., Kwon, H., . . . Son, H. (2010). Thyroglobulin antibody is associated with increased cancer risk in thyroid nodules. *Thyroid, 20*(8), 885-891.

Kohrle, J. (2000, Dec). The deiodinase family: selenoenzymes regulating thyroid hormone availability and action. *Cell. Mol. Life Sci., 57*(13-14), 1853-1863.

Koulouri, O., & Gurnell, M. (2013). How to interpret thyroid function tests. *13(3),* 282-286.

Krausz, A. E., Adler, B. L., Cabral, V., Navati, M., Doerner, J., Charafeddine, R. A., . . . Friedman, A. J. (2015). Curcumin-encapsulated nanoparticles as innovative antimicrobial and wound healing agent. *Nanomedicine, 11*(1), 195-206.

Lammers, K. M., Lu, R., Brownley, J., Lu, B., Gerard, C., Thomas, K., . . . Fasano, A. (2008). Gliadin Induces an Increase in Intestinal Permeability and Zonulin Release by Binding to the Chemokine Receptor CXCR3. *Gastroenterology, 135*(1), 194-204. Retrieved from https://www.ncbi.nlm.nih.gov/pmc/articles/PMC2653457/

Lechan, R. M., & Fekete, C. (2005). Role of thyroid hormone deiodination in the hypothalamus. *Thyroid, 15*(8), 883-897.

Lee, S. (2018, March 02). *Hashimoto Thyroiditis Workup*. Retrieved from Medscape: https://emedicine.medscape.com/article/120937-workup#c8

Lee, S., & Privalsky, M. L. (2005). Heterodimers of retinoic acid receptors and thyroid hormone receptors display unique combinatorial regulatory properties. *Mol. Endocrinol., 19*(4), 863-878.

Leoutsakos, V. (2004). A short history of the thyroid gland. *Hormones (Athens), 3*(4), 268-271.

Lerner, S. (2016, May 17). *New Evidence About the Dangers of Monsanto's Roundup*. Retrieved from The Intercept: https://theintercept.com/2016/05/17/new-evidence-about-the-dangers-of-monsantos-roundup/

Leschek, E; Cooper, DS. (2018, January 8). *Hashimoto's disease*. Retrieved from Office of Womens Health - U.S. Dept of Health and Human Services: https://www.womenshealth.gov/a-z-topics/hashimotos-disease

Lewis MD, C. A. (2013). *Enteroimmunology*. Carrabelle: Psy Press.

Lippi, G., Montagnana, M., Targher, G., Salvagno, G. L., & Guidi, G. C. (2008). Prevalence of Folic Acid and vitamin B12 deficiencies in patients with thyroid disorders. *Am. J. Med. Sci., 336*(1), 50-52.

Loos, C., Seppelt, R., Meier-Bethke, S., Schiemann, J., & Richter, O. (2003). Spatially explicit modelling of transgenic maize pollen dispersal and cross-pollination. *Journal of Theoretical Biology, 225*(2), 241-255. Retrieved from http://www.sciencedirect.com/science/article/pii/S002251 9303002431

Lord, R. S., & Bralley, J. (2012). *Laboratory Evaluations for Integrative and Functional Medicine, 2nd Ed.* Duluth: Genova Diagnostics.

Lowe, J. C. (2000). *The Metabolic Treatment of Fibromyalgia.* Boulder: McDowell Publishing Company.

Ma, J., & Li, X. (2015). Alteration in the cytokine levels and histopathological damage in common carp induced by glyphosate. *Chemosphere, 128,* 293-298.

Mangiapane, M. L., & Simpson, J. B. (1980). Subfornical organ: forebrain site of pressor and dipsogenic action of angiotensin II. *American Journal of Physiology-Regulatory, Integrative and Comparative Physiology, 239*(5), R382-R389. Retrieved from https://www.physiology.org/doi/10.1152/ajpregu.1980.239.5.R382

Marques, C. D., Dantas, A. T., Fragoso, T. S., & Duarte, A. L. (2010). The importance of vitamin D levels in autoimmune diseases. *Revista Brasileira de Reumatologia, 50*(1), 67-80. Retrieved from http://www.scielo.br/scielo.php?script=sci_abstract&pid=S0482-50042010000100007&lng=en&nrm=iso&tlng=en

Master John, C. (2011, October 13). *Wheat Belly - The Toll of Hubris on Human Health.* Retrieved from Chris Master John, PhD: https://chrismasterjohnphd.com/2011/10/13/wheat-belly-toll-of-hubris-on-human/

Mazzone, G., D'Argenio, G., Lembo, V., Vitaglione, P., Vitiello, R., Loperto, I., . . . Caporaso, N. (2013). Decaffeinated Coffee Reduces Intestinal Leakiness in Rats Fed With a HFD by Modulating Occludin and Zonulin-1 Expression. *Gastroenterology, 144*(5), S-1021. Retrieved from http://www.gastrojournal.org/article/S0016-5085(13)63791-9/fulltext

McAninch, E. A., & Bianco, A. C. (2016). The History and Future of Treatment of Hypothyroidism. *Ann Intern Med, 164*(1), 50-56. Retrieved from https://www.ncbi.nlm.nih.gov/pmc/articles/PMC4980994/

McCall, K. A., Huang, C.-c., & Fierke, C. A. (2000). Function and Mechanism of Zinc Metalloenzymes. *J Nutr, 130*(5), 1437S--1446S. Retrieved from https://academic.oup.com/jn/article/130/5/1437S/4686409

McMillan, M., Spinks, E. A., & Fenwick, G. R. (1986). Preliminary observations on the effect of dietary brussels sprouts on thyroid function. *Hum Toxicol, 5*(1), 15-19.

Mesnage, R., & Antoniou, M. N. (2017). Facts and Fallacies in the Debate on Glyphosate Toxicity. *Front Public Health, 5,* 316.

Meyer, N., & Reguant-Closa, A. (2017). Eat as If You Could Save the Planet and Win!: Sustainability Integration into Nutrition for Exercise and Sport. *Nutrients, 9*(4), 412.

Mink, P. J., Mandel, J. S., Lundin, J. I., & Sceurman, B. K. (2011). Epidemiologic studies of glyphosate and non-cancer health outcomes: a review. *Regul. Toxicol. Pharmacol., 61*(2), 172-184.

Molnar, I., Balazs, C., Szegedi, G., & Sipka, S. (2002). Inhibition of type 2,5'-deiodinase by tumor necrosis factor alpha, interleukin-6 and interferon gamma in human thyroid tissue. *Immunol. Lett., 80*(1), 3-7.

Moran, C., & Chatterjee, K. (2015). Resistance to thyroid hormone due to defective thyroid receptor alpha. *Best Pract Res Clin Endocrinol Metab, 29*(4), 647-657. Retrieved from https://www.ncbi.nlm.nih.gov/pmc/articles/PMC4559105/

Morley, J. E., Gordon, J., & Hershman, J. M. (1980). Zinc deficiency, chronic starvation, and hypothalamic-pituitary-thyroid function. *Am. J. Clin. Nutr., 33*(8), 1767-1770.

Moss, M. (2013, February 26). *How The Food Industry Manipulates Taste Buds With 'Salt Sugar Fat'.* Retrieved from NPR: https://www.npr.org/sections/thesalt/2013/02/26/172969

363/how-the-food-industry-manipulates-taste-buds-with-salt-sugar-fat

Moss, M. (2013, February 24). *The Extraordinary Science of Addictive Junk Food*. Retrieved from New York Times: https://www.nytimes.com/2013/02/24/magazine/the-extraordinary-science-of-junk-food.html

Munoz-Torres, M., Varsavsky, M., & Alonso, G. (2006). Lactose intolerance revealed by severe resistance to treatment with levothyroxine. *Thyroid, 16*(11), 1171-1173.

Mussig, K., Thamer, C., Bares, R., Lipp, H.-P., Haring, H.-U., & Gallwitz, B. (2006). Iodine-Induced Thyrotoxicosis After Ingestion of Kelp-Containing Tea. *J Gen Intern Med, 21*(6), C11-C14. Retrieved from https://www.ncbi.nlm.nih.gov/pmc/articles/PMC1924637/

Myers, J. P., Antoniou, M. N., Blumberg, B., Carroll, L., Colborn, T., Everett, L. G., . . . Benbrook, C. M. (2016). Concerns over use of glyphosate-based herbicides and risks associated with exposures: a consensus statement. *Environmental Health, 15*, 19. Retrieved from https://doi.org/10.1186/s12940-016-0117-0

Nanan, R., & Wall, J. R. (2010). Remission of Hashimoto's thyroiditis in a twelve-year-old girl with thyroid changes documented by ultrasonography. *Thyroid, 20*(10), 1187-1190.

National Institutes of Health. (2006, October 19). *Dandelion*. Retrieved from National Center for Complementary and Interative Health: https://nccih.nih.gov/health/dandelion

Negro, R. (2008). Selenium and thyroid autoimmunity. *Biologics, 2*(2), 265-273. Retrieved from https://www.ncbi.nlm.nih.gov/pmc/articles/PMC2721352/

Niazi, A., Kalra, S., Irfan, A., & Islam, A. (2011). Thyroidology over the ages. *Indian J Endocrinol Metab, 15*(Suppl2), S121-S126.

Retrieved from
https://www.ncbi.nlm.nih.gov/pmc/articles/PMC3169859/

Nierenberg, A. A., Fava, M., Trivedi, M. H., Wisniewski, S. R., Thase, M. E., McGrath, P. J., . . . Rush, A. J. (2006). A comparison of lithium and T(3) augmentation following two failed medication treatments for depression: a STAR*D report. *Am J Psychiatry, 163*(9), 1519--1530; quiz 1665.

Noureldine, S. I., & Tufano, R. P. (2015). Association of Hashimoto's thyroiditis and thyroid cancer. *Curr Opin Oncol, 27*(1), 21-25.

Ogiwara, T., Araki, O., Morimura, T., Tsunekawa, K., Mori, M., & Murakami, M. (2013). A novel mechanism for the inhibition of type 2 iodothyronine deiodinase by tumor necrosis factor alpha: involvement of proteasomal degradation. *Endocr. J., 60*(9), 1035-1045.

Ongphiphadhanakul, B., Fang, S. L., Tang, K. T., Patwardhan, N. A., & Braverman, L. E. (1994). Tumor necrosis factor-alpha decreases thyrotropin-induced 5'-deiodinase activity in FRTL-5 thyroid cells. *Eur. J. Endocrinol., 130*(5), 502-507.

Ortiga-Carvalho, T. M., Chiamolera, M. I., Pazos-Moura, C. C., & Wondisford, F. E. (2016). Hypothalamus-Pituitary-Thyroid Axis. *Compr Physiol, 6*(3), 1387-1428.

OSU. (2014, October). *Supplemental Forms of Vitamin C*. Retrieved from Linus Pauling Institute Oregon State University: http://lpi.oregonstate.edu/mic/vitamins/vitamin-C/supplemental-forms

PAN Staff. (2009 , May 13). *Pesticides on Wheat Flour*. Retrieved from What's On My Food: http://www.whatsonmyfood.org/food.jsp?food=WF

Panda, S., & Kar, A. (1998). Changes in thyroid hormone concentrations after administration of ashwagandha root extract to adult male mice. *J. Pharm. Pharmacol., 50*(9), 1065-1068.

Pang, X., Hershman, J., & M. C. (1989). Impairment of hypothalamic-pituitary-thyroid function in rats treated with human recombinant tumor necrosis factor-alpha (cachectin). *Endocrinology*, 76-84. Retrieved from https://www.ncbi.nlm.nih.gov/pubmed/2500334

Parish, M. (2006, February 21). *How do salt and sugar prevent microbial spoilage?* Retrieved from Scientic American: https://www.scientificamerican.com/article/how-do-salt-and-sugar-pre/

Patel, B., Schutte, R., Sporns, P., Doyle, J., Jewel, L., & Fedorak, R. N. (2002). Potato glycoalkaloids adversely affect intestinal permeability and aggravate inflammatory bowel disease. *Inflamm. Bowel Dis., 8*(5), 340-346.

Pekary, A. E., Lukaski, H. C., Mena, I., & Hershman, J. M. (1991). Processing of TRH precursor peptides in rat brain and pituitary is zinc dependent. *Peptides, 12*(5), 1025-1032.

Perrild, H., Hansen, J. M., Skovsted, L., & Christensen, L. K. (1983). Different effects of propranolol, alprenolol, sotalol, atenolol and metoprolol on serum T3 and serum rT3 in hyperthyroidism. *Clin. Endocrinol. (Oxf), 18*(2), 139-142.

Pessione, E. (2012). Lactic acid bacteria contribution to gut microbiota complexity: lights and shadows. *Front Cell Infect Microbiol, 2*, 86.

Peterson, S. J., McAninch, E. A., & Bianco, A. C. (2016). Is a Normal TSH Synonymous With "Euthyroidism" in Levothyroxine Monotherapy? *J. Clin. Endocrinol. Metab., 101*(12), 4964-4973.

Pol, C. J., Muller, A., Zuidwijk, M. J., van Deel, E. D., Kaptein, E., Saba, A., . . . Simonides, W. S. (2011). Left-ventricular remodeling after myocardial infarction is associated with a cardiomyocyte-specific hypothyroid condition. *Endocrinology, 152*(2), 669-679.

Potential effects of agrochemicals in Argentina. (2013, October 21). Retrieved from Boston.com: http://archive.boston.com/bigpicture/2013/10/agrochemic al_spraying_in_argen.html

Publishing, Harvard Health. (2011, June 1). *Cut salt - it won't affect your iodine intake.* Retrieved from Harvard Health: https://www.health.harvard.edu/heart-health/cut-salt-it-wont-affect-your-iodine-intake

Pyzik, A., Grywalska, E., Matyjaszek-Matuszek, B., & RoliÅ„ski, J. (2015). Immune Disorders in Hashimoto's Thyroiditis: What Do We Know So Far? *J Immunol Res, 2015*, 979167. Retrieved from https://www.ncbi.nlm.nih.gov/pmc/articles/PMC4426893/

Ramadan, G., Al-Kahtani, M. A., & El-Sayed, W. M. (2011). Anti-inflammatory and anti-oxidant properties of Curcuma longa (turmeric) versus Zingiber officinale (ginger) rhizomes in rat adjuvant-induced arthritis. *Inflammation, 34*(4), 291-301.

Rashid, T., & Ebringer, A. (2012). Autoimmunity in Rheumatic Diseases Is Induced by Microbial Infections via Crossreactivity or Molecular Mimicry. *Autoimmune Diseases.* Retrieved from https://www.hindawi.com/journals/ad/2012/539282/abs/

Rashid, T., Wilson, C., & Ebringer, A. (2013). The Link between Ankylosing Spondylitis, Crohn's Disease, Klebsiella, and Starch Consumption. *Clin Dev Immunol, 2013.* Retrieved from https://www.ncbi.nlm.nih.gov/pmc/articles/PMC3678459/

Raval-Pandya, M., Freedman, L. P., Li, H., & Christakos, S. (1998). Thyroid hormone receptor does not heterodimerize with the vitamin D receptor but represses vitamin D receptor-mediated transactivation. *Mol. Endocrinol., 12*(9), 1367-1379.

Rayman, M. P. (2000). The importance of selenium to human health. *Lancet, 356*(9225), 233-241.

Rayman, M. P. (2012). Selenium and human health. *Lancet, 379*(9822), 1256-1268.

Reuters Staff. (2010, February 12). *Underactive thyroid linked to pesticide exposure.* Retrieved from Reuters: https://www.reuters.com/article/us-underactive-thyroid/underactive-thyroid-linked-to-pesticide-exposure-idUSTRE61B54U20100212

Richman, E. L., Carroll, P. R., & Chan, J. M. (2012). Vegetable and fruit intake after diagnosis and risk of prostate cancer progression. *Int. J. Cancer, 131*(1), 201-210.

Rogers, N. M., Kireta, S., & Coates, P. T. (2010). Curcumin induces maturation-arrested dendritic cells that expand regulatory T cells in vitro and in vivo. *Clin. Exp. Immunol., 162*(3), 460-473.

Rubio-Tapia, A., Kyle, R. A., Kaplan, E. L., Johnson, D. R., Page, W., Erdtmann, F., . . . Murray, J. A. (2009). Increased prevalence and mortality in undiagnosed celiac disease. *Gastroenterology, 137*(1), 88-93.

RX List Editor. (2018, March 01). *Thyrolar (Liotrix): Side Effects, Interactions, Warning, Dosage & Uses.* Retrieved from RX List: https://www.rxlist.com/thyrolar-drug.htm#description

Saad, M. J., Morais, S. L., & Saad, S. T. (1991). Reduced cortisol secretion in patients with iron deficiency. *Ann. Nutr. Metab., 35*(2), 111-115.

Samsel, A., & Seneff, S. (2013). Glyphosate, pathways to modern diseases II: Celiac sprue and gluten intolerance. *Interdiscip Toxicol, 6*(4), 159-184.

Saranac, L., Zivanovic, S., Bjelakovic, B., Stamenkovic, H., Novak, M., & Kamenov, B. (2011). Why is the thyroid so prone to autoimmune disease? *Horm Res Paediatr, 75*(3), 157-165.

Schomburg, L. (2016). Dietary Selenium and Human Health. *Nutrients, 9*(1), 22. Retrieved from https://www.ncbi.nlm.nih.gov/pmc/articles/PMC5295066/

Seaborg, E. (2016, January 8). *Beware of Biotin.* Retrieved from Endocrine News: https://endocrinenews.endocrine.org/january-2016-thyroid-month-beware-of-biotin/

Sharp, R. (2012, October 15). *Americans Eat Their Weight in Genetically Engineered Food.* Retrieved from Environmental Working Group: https://www.ewg.org/agmag/2012/10/americans-eat-their-weight-genetically-engineered-food

Sheer, R., & Moss, D. (2011, March 12). *Are There Links between Pesticides and Other Chemicals to Thyroid Disease?* Retrieved from Scientific American: https://www.scientificamerican.com/article/pesticide-use-thyroid-disease/

Shehata, A., Schrodl, W., Aldin, A., Hafez, H., & Kruger, M. (2013). The effect of glyphosate on potential pathogens and beneficial members of poultry microbiota in vitro. *Curr. Microbiol., 66*(4), 350-358.

Shewry, P. R. (2009). Wheat. *J Exp Bot, 60*(6), 1537-1553. Retrieved from https://academic.oup.com/jxb/article/60/6/1537/517393

Shoba, G., Joy, D., Joseph, T., Majeed, M., Rajendran, R., & Srinivas, P. S. (1998). Influence of piperine on the pharmacokinetics of curcumin in animals and human volunteers. *Planta Med., 64*(4), 353-356.

Siddiqi, M. A., Laessig, R. H., & Reed, K. D. (2003). Polybrominated diphenyl ethers (PBDEs): new pollutants-old diseases. *Clin Med Res, 1*(4), 281-290.

Sinha, R., Sinha, I., Calcagnotto, A., Trushin, N., Haley, J. S., Schell, T. D., & Richie, J. P. (2018). Oral supplementation with liposomal glutathione elevates body stores of glutathione and markers of immune function. *Eur J Clin Nutr, 72*(1), 105-111.

Smith, J. (2018, March 15). *Non-GMO Shopping Guide.* Retrieved from Non-GMO Shopping Guide: http://www.nongmoshoppingguide.com/

Song, S., & Oka, T. (2003). Regulation of type II deiodinase expression by EGF and glucocorticoid in HC11 mouse mammary epithelium. *Am. J. Physiol. Endocrinol. Metab., 284*(6), E1119-1124.

Souza, L. L., Nunes, M. O., Paula, G. S., Cordeiro, A., Penha-Pinto, V., Neto, J. F., . . . Pazos-Moura, C. C. (2010). Effects of dietary fish oil on thyroid hormone signaling in the liver. *J. Nutr. Biochem., 21*(10), 935-940.

Spangnoli Gabardi, C. (2015, December). *The Dangers of Glyphosate: From Glucose Intolerance to Cancer.* Retrieved from Eluxe Magazine: http://eluxemagazine.com/magazine/dangers-of-glyphosate/

Stansbury ND, J. (2016). Adrenal and Thyroid Modulation with Botanical Medicine. *AARM Restorative Medicine Regional Conference* (pp. 47-70). Vancouver: Association for the Advancement of Restorative Medicine.

Starr, M. (2005). *Hypothyroidism Type 2: The Epidemic.* Columbus: Mark Start Trust.

Steve Plogsted, P. (2018, 03 30). *New Gluten-Free Drug List.* Retrieved from Gluten Free Drugs: http://www.glutenfreedrugs.com/newlist.htm

Sugawara, M., Kita, T., Lee, E. D., Takamatsu, J., Hagen, G. A., Kuma, K., & Medeiros-Neto, G. A. (1988). Deficiency of superoxide dismutase in endemic goiter tissue. *J. Clin. Endocrinol. Metab., 67*(6), 1156-1161.

Tagami, T., Park, Y., & Jameson, J. L. (1999). Mechanisms that mediate negative regulation of the thyroid-stimulating hormone alpha gene by the thyroid hormone receptor. *J. Biol. Chem., 274*(32), 22345-22353.

Takasu, N., Komiya, I., Asawa, T., Nagasawa, Y., & Yamada, T. (1990). Test for recovery from hypothyroidism during thyroxine therapy in Hashimoto's thyroiditis. *Lancet, 336*(8723), 1084-1086.

Turner, B. (2015, July 28). *Is American wheat different than European wheat?* Retrieved from Howstuffworks: https://recipes.howstuffworks.com/is-american-wheat-different-than-european-wheat.htm

U.S. Food and Drug Administration. (2017, December 1). *Current and Resolved Drug Shortages and Discontinuations Reported to FDA.* Retrieved from U.S. Food and Drug Administration: https://www.accessdata.fda.gov/scripts/drugshortages/dsp_ActiveIngredientDetails.cfm?AI=Liotrix%20(Thyrolar)%20Tablets&st=c&tab=tabs-1

Vasiluk, L., Pinto, L. J., & Moore, M. M. (2005). Oral bioavailability of glyphosate: studies using two intestinal cell lines. *Environ. Toxicol. Chem., 24*(1), 153-160.

Vasquez, A. (2014). *Textbook of Clinical Nutrition and Functional Medicine, vol. 1: Essential Knowledge for Safe Action and Effective Treatment (Inflammation Mastery & Functional Inflammology).* Barcelona: International College of Human Nutrition and Functional Medicine.

Vasquez, A. (2015). *Human Microbiome and Dysbiosis in Clinical Disease: Volume 1: Parts 1 - 4*. Portland: International College of Human Nutrition and Functional Medicine.

Verloop, H., Dekkers, O. M., Peeters, R. P., Schoones, J. W., & Smit, J. W. (2014). Genetics in endocrinology: genetic variation in deiodinases: a systematic review of potential clinical effects in humans. *Eur. J. Endocrinol., 171*(3), R123-135.

Vierhapper, H., Grubeck-Loebenstein, B., Ferenci, P., Lochs, H., Bratusch-Marrain, P., & Waldhausl, W. (1981). Alterations in thyroxine metabolism in Crohn's disease. *Hepatogastroenterology, 28*(1), 31-33.

Wahlstrom, B., & Blennow, G. (1978). A study on the fate of curcumin in the rat. *Acta Pharmacol Toxicol (Copenh), 43*(2), 86-92.

Wajner, S. M., Goemann, I. M., Bueno, A. L., Larsen, P. R., & Maia, A. L. (2011). IL-6 promotes nonthyroidal illness syndrome by blocking thyroxine activation while promoting thyroid hormone inactivation in human cells. *J. Clin. Invest., 121*(5), 1834-1845.

Wajner, S. M., Rohenkohl, H. C., Serrano, T., & Maia, A. L. (2015). Sodium selenite supplementation does not fully restore oxidative stress-induced deiodinase dysfunction: {Implications} for the nonthyroidal illness syndrome. *Redox Biol, 6*, 436-445.

Water, J. V., Ishibashi, H., Coppel, R. L., & Gershwin, M. E. (2001). Molecular mimicry and primary biliary cirrhosis: Premises not promises. *Hepatology, 33*(4), 771-775. Retrieved from https://aasldpubs.onlinelibrary.wiley.com/doi/abs/10.1053/jhep.2001.23902

Weiss, R. E., Dumitrescu, A., & Refetoff, S. (2010). Approach to the Patient with Resistance to Thyroid Hormone and Pregnancy.

J Clin Endocrinol Metab, 95(7), 3094-3102. Retrieved from https://www.ncbi.nlm.nih.gov/pmc/articles/PMC2928892/

Wentz, I. (2013). *Hashimoto's Thyroiditis: Lifestyle Interventions for Finding and Treating the Root Cause.* Chicago: Wentz, LLC.

Wilson, D. (2013, March 28). *Guggul is an herb that supports thyroid health.* Retrieved from Wilson's Tempurature Syndrome: http://www.wilsonssyndrome.com/guggul-is-an-herb-that-supports-thyroid-health/

Wilson, D. (2016). Sub Laboratory Hypothyroidism and it Emperical Use of T3. *AARM Restorative Medicine Regional Conference* (pp. 26-33). Vancouver: Association for the Advancement of Restorative Medicine.

Wilson, J. L. (2001). *Adrenal Fatigue: The 21st Century Stress Syndrome.* Seattle: Smart Publications.

Zava, T. T., & Zava, D. T. (2011). Assessment of Japanese iodine intake based on seaweed consumption in Japan: A literature-based analysis. *Thyroid Research, 4,* 14. Retrieved from https://doi.org/10.1186/1756-6614-4-14

Zdilla, M. J., Starkey, L. D., & Saling, J. R. (2015). A Taste-intensity Visual Analog Scale: An Improved Zinc Taste-test Protocol. *Integr Med (Encinitas), 14*(2), 34-38. Retrieved from https://www.ncbi.nlm.nih.gov/pmc/articles/PMC4566477/

Zhu, L., Bai, X., Teng, W.-p., Shan, Z.-y., Wang, W.-w., Fan, C.-l., . . . Zhang, H.-m. (2012). Effects of selenium supplementation on antibodies of autoimmune thyroiditis. *Zhonghua Yi Xue Za Zhi, 92*(32), 2256-2260.

Zimmermann, M. (2007). Interactions of Vitamin A and Iodine Deficiencies: Effects on the Pituitary-Thyroid Axis. *International Journal for Vitamin and Nutrition Research, 77*(3), 236-240. Retrieved from https://econtent.hogrefe.com/doi/abs/10.1024/0300-9831.77.3.236

Zimmermann, M. B. (2009). Iodine deficiency. *Endocr. Rev., 30*(4), 376-408.

Zimmermann, M. B., Wegmeller, R., Zeder, C., Chaouki, N., & Torresani, T. (2004). The Effects of Vitamin A Deficiency and Vitamin A Supplementation on Thyroid Function in Goitrous Children. *J Clin Endocrinol Metab, 89*(11), 5441-5447. Retrieved from https://academic.oup.com/jcem/article/89/11/5441/2844339

Zimmermann, M., & Kohrle, J. (2002). The impact of iron and selenium deficiencies on iodine and thyroid metabolism: biochemistry and relevance to public health. *Thyroid, 12*(10), 867-878.

ABOUT THE AUTHOR

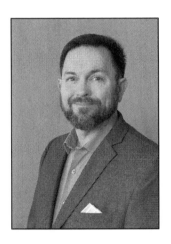

Dr. Shawn Soszka is a naturopathic physician, functional medicine practitioner, and licensed acupuncturist who has used a holistic approach to treat thyroid conditions effectively for nearly 20 years. He has helped thousands of patients restore their health and improve quality of life.

This book includes bonus videos and materials to help you fix your thyroid. Get them at:
www.TheThyroidFixBook.com/bonuses.

Made in the USA
Columbia, SC
02 May 2018